# Recover Smarter

*The Ultimate Guide to Healing After Surgery*

Kevin Rebman

Method & Myth Media—Minneapolis, MN
ISBN: 979-8-9989964-0-5
Library of Congress Control Number: 2025910886
Title: *Recover Smarter: The Ultimate Guide to Healing After Surgery*
Author: Kevin Rebman, *BCTMB, AAS, BA, MS, NREMT*
Digital distribution | 2025
Paperback | 2025

Published in the United States by New Book Authors Publishing

# Dedication

This book is dedicated to those who are courageously navigating the journey of recovery, either voluntarily or by some other circumstance. May this guide empower you to reclaim your strength, rediscover your confidence in your body, and embrace the healing process with hope and clarity.

*"If you're going through recovery, keep going, but feel free to complain quietly along the way."*

~ Nora Ephron—Screenwriter, Director, Journalist.

# Table of Contents

# Preface

When I first began working with post-surgical patients as a clinical massage therapist, I didn't set out to write a book. I set out to solve a problem. Why are patients not prepared for successful recovery from the start?

As more and more patients came to see me for clinical manual soft tissue therapy (clinical massage) weeks, sometimes months, after their procedure, they were frustrated, swollen, resigned, and disheartened with the results. The patients lacked information from their healthcare team, so mistakenly, they turned to Facebook and Google for the answers. Assured by their doctor and nurses they would recover in a certain timeframe, that milestone came and went, but they didn't feel "normal" yet.

Patients tell me "What did I do wrong? I don't look like the before-and-after photos in the brochure." They had hard lumps, tightness in their incisions and surgical area, fatigue from 'fighting' their recovery, and limited range of motion. Most notable was the fact they had *questions which no one had answered.* Why not?

Patients were not set up to succeed in recovery, and that is not right. Surgeons are fantastically talented at fixing things, but once the surgery is over, many have nothing more to offer unless something bad happens. Recovery is often treated as an afterthought, just a passive activity. Guidance I hear is – just hang out, walk a bit, compress here and there, maybe start physical therapy in 4-6 weeks. Well, recovery, like everything else in this world, requires effort and attention to details.

Post-surgical recovery is an *active effort* and needs daily attention! Patients should not blame themselves for not knowing what to do.

My advice: Don't give up on your recovery outcomes!

**From Clinical Massage to Recovery Partner**

I own a clinical manual soft tissue clinic called Return to Play Institute, LLC in Minneapolis, MN. We specialize in clinical manual soft tissue therapy – also known as medical massage and rehabilitation. I use every bit of knowledge from my training in lymphatic drainage, decongestive therapy, oncology massage, scar tissue therapy, wound care, gross anatomy, and neuromuscular therapy to bring a comprehensive toolkit to each patient treatment. These patients are recovering from trauma, surgery, and overuse. One client called us "muscle doc's." We bridge the gap between surgery and true recovery, working alongside plastic surgeons, orthopedic doctors, and physical therapists to offer care that picks up where the hospital discharge ends.

My team has helped people bounce back from breast reconstruction, tummy tucks, ACL repairs, BBLs, liposuctions, gender-affirming procedures, spinal surgeries, thigh lifts, and countless other surgical procedures. Some were elective, some weren't. But all had one thing in common: the patient wanted to heal fully, not just *functionally*, but **comfortably, confidently, and completely**.

Over the past several years, I've learned what worked, and what didn't. We saw patterns in pain, swelling, and scar tissue formation and reduction. We tested tissue manipulation techniques. We reviewed research. And most importantly, we *listened*, to our clients, to their frustrations, and to their successes!

This book brings much of that information together into one comprehensive resource.

**Why I Wrote This Book**

This book exists because I wanted to give you, the reader, the same level of insight, encouragement, and support that our in-person clients receive at Return to Play Institute (RTPI) in Minneapolis.

You deserve to know:

- what's happening inside the body at each healing stage

- what you can do to speed recovery, reduce complications, and optimize results
- which products, supplements, and techniques are truly useful, and which are just hype
- how to prepare your home, mindset, and body *before* surgery so you're not scrambling afterward
- how to interpret symptoms like swelling, tightness, or scar changes without panic

Most importantly, you deserve to feel empowered, not confused, about your recovery.

This book is here to help you heal *smarter*, not harder.

**What This Book Is and Is Not**

This book is:

- a research-backed, easy-to-understand manual for post-surgical healing
- a roadmap based on both clinical experience and modern medical insights
- a holistic guide that includes nutrition, mindset, mobility, and manual therapy
- designed for patients and their caregivers, but useful to professionals, too

This book is ***not***:

- a substitute for your surgeon's directions. Every surgery and every body is different. This book is meant to complement your medical care, not replace it. Use it in partnership with your providers.

- a self-care massage manuscript. This book is not going to teach you manual lymphatic drainage or scar tissue homework – both of those are best learned from your local, well-trained, certified medical massage therapist. Facebook, YouTube and TikTok are full of bad instruction, so learn it in person from a pro.

- a book filled with vague advice or miracle promises. Recovery is real work. There are ups and downs. Some parts of recovery will be frustrating. Some will be amazing. But through it all, you'll be better equipped with this book by your side.

**How to Use This Book**

You can read this book cover to cover or skip around to the chapters that speak to your current stage. It is organized it by both recovery *phases* and key *topics*. You'll find:

- **Pre-Surgery Prep**: how to optimize nutrition, sleep, and mobility before going under the knife
- **Recovery Phases**: a breakdown of what to expect week by week, including the hemostasis, inflammatory, proliferation, and remodeling stages
- **Swelling & Inflammation**: how to manage fluid retention, bruising, and tissue trauma
- **Scar Management**: insights on tissue remodeling, products, manipulation techniques, and how to reduce visible scarring
- **Nutrition & Supplementation**: evidence-based guidance on what to eat and what to avoid, including key supplements like turmeric and collagen
- **Manual Therapy & Movement**: when to start massage or mobility work, how to do it safely, and why it matters
- **Emotional Health**: tips to stay grounded, calm, and focused through this emotionally vulnerable period

You'll also find checklists, symptoms to watch for, and gentle reminders that *progress is not always linear, and that's okay.*

**Who This Book Is For**

This book is for you, the patient undergoing surgery, from minor cosmetic tweaks to major orthopedic or reconstructive work. This book is also for caregivers, family members, and healthcare professionals who want to support recovery more effectively.

Whether you're an athlete recovering from a torn ligament, a parent bouncing back from a C-section, a patient preparing for a mastectomy, or someone simply seeking a smoother cosmetic surgery journey, this book is written for *you*.

**Final Thoughts**

To recover well, you don't have to know all the answers. You just need the right guidance, and the willingness to follow through.

You'll find both here.

No one should feel lost, scared, or alone during surgery recovery. My goal, with this book, is that you feel prepared, informed, and in control of your healing process. I hope that one day you'll look back on your recovery journey, as something you conquered in a transformative, empowering way. Your recovery is now part of your story!

Wishing you a smooth recovery, strong outcomes, and feeling like yourself again, maybe even better!

In Health,
**Kevin Rebman, BCTMB, AAS, BA, MS, NREMT**
Board Certified Therapist in Massage and Bodywork
Clinical Myotherapist & Founder
Return to Play Institute, LLC
*"Feel better. Recover quicker. Return to Play faster!"*
Minneapolis, MN, USA

# Introduction

## Why Recovery Matters after Surgery

Surgery is more than just an aesthetic transformation or removal of parts, or replacement of a joint; it is a medical procedure that requires a well-structured recovery plan to achieve the best possible results. Recovery is crucial with all surgical procedures that involve trauma to the body. Knee and hip replacements, injury repair surgeries, C-sections, and reconstructive surgeries following cancer treatments. In all cases, the body must undergo an intensive healing process that requires proper care, time, and attention.

We often hear of athletes who recover from a career-ending surgery in a record time – better than expected. Why did they recover faster? How did they do it?

The short answer is - informed decisions, perseverance, and they, themselves, took an active role in their recovery plan. Yes, they had a great recovery team, but the real work must be done by the patient.

## The Science Behind Recovery

Surgical procedures create controlled trauma to the body. As a response, the body initiates a healing process that involves inflammation, tissue remodeling, and scar formation (Gurtner et al., 2011). Recovery is not simply about resting; it is a complex biological process that involves immune function, circulation, lymphatic drainage, and wound healing. Ignoring post-operative care can result in prolonged swelling, infection, poor scar formation, and range of motion issues.

For orthopedic surgeries like knee and hip replacements, post-operative rehabilitation is essential to restore mobility, reduce swelling, and prevent complications such as deep vein thrombosis (DVT). Similarly, in C-sections, proper incision care and core muscle rehabilitation play a critical role in long-term recovery. For patients undergoing reconstructive surgery, wound healing, lymphatic function, and scar management are essential for optimal outcomes. Regardless of the type of surgery, recovery plays a pivotal role in determining the success of the procedure and overall patient well-being.

Studies show that patients who adhere to post-operative recovery protocols experience faster healing times, fewer complications, and improved surgical outcomes (Mustoe et al., 2002). By following expert-recommended care strategies, patients can significantly enhance their results and minimize risks.

Discussions in this book will focus on many surgeries – they all require a recovery protocol based on the type of trauma placed on body by the medical procedure.

A well-structured recovery plan is required to achieve the best possible results. Whether you are undergoing a knee replacement, facelift, liposuction, a tummy tuck, or breast reconstruction, your body needs time to heal properly. Understanding the importance of recovery and how to optimize it can make the difference between a smooth healing process and unnecessary complications.

## Common Misconceptions About Recovery

Many patients mistakenly believe that recovery is a passive process, where simply avoiding physical exertion is enough. However, active participation in recovery, such as proper wound care, nutrition, and controlled movement, can significantly impact healing. Other misconceptions include:

- **"Pain equals healing."** Pain is a natural part of recovery, but excessive pain can be a sign of complications like hematomas or infection (Reid et al., 2015).

- **"Bruising and swelling are the same."** While both are common post-surgery, swelling results from fluid buildup and inflammation, whereas bruising is caused by small blood vessel leaks (Atiyeh et al., 2015).
- **"Scarring is ugly and unavoidable."** Proper scar management, including silicone treatments and hydration, can drastically reduce scar formation (O'Brien & Jones, 2013).

## What to Expect from This Book

This book is designed to provide **comprehensive, evidence-based strategies** to help you recover safely and efficiently. Each chapter will cover distinct aspects of post-operative care, offering actionable advice backed by medical research.

## Key Topics Covered

- **Understanding Cosmetic Surgery Recovery**: The phases of healing and why recovery varies by procedure.
- **Preparing for Surgery**: How to optimize your body and home environment for a smoother post-operative experience.
- **Managing Swelling and Bruising**: Understanding how to reduce post-surgical inflammation using lymphatic drainage, hydration, and compression.
- **Wound Care and Scar Prevention**: The best methods to clean incisions, prevent infections, and reduce scarring.
- **Lymphatic Health and Drainage**: How the lymphatic system affects healing and why manual lymphatic drainage (MLD) is critical for recovery.
- **Nutrition for Optimal Healing**: The role of vitamins, hydration, and anti-inflammatory foods in post-operative recovery.
- **Activity and Movement**: How to safely reintroduce movement and prevent complications like blood clots.

- **Mental Health & Emotional Recovery**: Coping with body changes, post-op emotions, and stress management techniques.
- **Long-Term Maintenance and Beauty Tips**: Maintaining surgical results, skincare routines, and when to consider revision surgery.

This book aims to **empower patients** (you) with knowledge, enabling them to take an active role in their recovery. By following the principles outlined in this book, you can maximize your healing potential and enjoy the best possible results from your procedure.

## Disclaimer

This book is not intended to serve as medical direction, nor should it replace advice from a qualified medical professional. Patients should always consult their surgeon or primary care provider regarding their specific post-operative care. This book is based on best practices in post-operative recovery. The information provided is educational and should not be considered a substitute for personalized medical guidance.

## Encouraging Further Research

Thomas J. Watson, founder of IBM once said: *"The ability to ask the right question is more than half the battle of finding the answer."*

While it is easy to post a question on the Internet, beware of the answers received! Patients are encouraged to take an active role in their recovery by conducting their own research on post-operative care. Knowledge in the medical field continues to evolve. Patients should utilize reputable sources such as the **National Institutes of Health (NIH)**, **peer-reviewed medical journals**, and **professional healthcare organizations** to further their understanding of the topics presented here. Being well-informed empowers you to make the best decisions regarding your recovery and long-term health.

# Chapter 1

Understanding Stages of Surgery Recovery

Surgical recovery is more than just a physical process, it's a journey that touches every aspect of a person's life. Whether you are recovering from a facelift or healing after a C-section, your body follows a remarkably consistent sequence of healing. Understanding the stages of recovery not only helps you feel more in control but also empowers you to make better decisions about your care.

## The Healing Process: Stages of Recovery

Each stage is marked by distinct biological changes, and while these stages follow a general timeline, they can vary widely depending on your procedure, overall health, and adherence to aftercare protocols. Recovery is not linear, and your body may take two steps forward and one step back. That is normal, and part of the healing rhythm.

### Stage 1: Hemostasis (Immediately Post-Surgery)

As soon as your surgery ends, your body kicks into survival mode. Blood vessels constrict to reduce bleeding, and platelets rush in to form a clot over the surgical site. This clot is more than just a bandage; it serves as a scaffolding for the healing process to begin. It also helps seal the area from bacteria, reducing the risk of infection.

At this stage, you may notice some mild oozing at the incision site. This is expected, but anything more than light spotting should be discussed with your surgeon. Minimizing movement and keeping the wound covered are critical. It is like setting the foundation for a house, if it shifts too soon, the rest of the structure cannot hold.

### Stage 2: Inflammation (1–5 Days Post-Surgery)

Inflammation often gets a bad rap, but in this case, it is a good thing, at least initially. Your immune system sends in white blood cells to clean the area of damaged cells and potential invaders. You will see swelling, redness, and feel some warmth around the surgical site. That is your body at work.

Pain or tenderness is common here, too, and it is not just in your head. Inflammatory molecules like histamines and cytokines increase sensitivity in nerve endings. Compression garments, if approved, can help reduce this inflammation, and manual lymphatic drainage has shown to support lymphatic function and decrease edema (Atiyeh et al., 2015). During this phase, monitoring for signs of infection, like increased redness, fever, or foul-smelling discharge, is crucial.

### Stage 3: Proliferation (5–21 Days Post-Surgery)

This is when the heavy lifting happens. Your body begins rebuilding the damaged area, laying down collagen and new blood vessels. While phagocytes, a type of white blood cell, are busy engulfing and removing dead and damaged cells in the surgery area, fibroblast cells secrete collagen proteins, the materials your skin and tissue need to repair. You may notice scabs, tightness, or even itching, which is often a good sign.

Supporting your body's efforts here is essential. A diet rich in protein, vitamin C, and hydration fuels the collagen-building process (Mustoe et al., 2002). Light, guided movement can encourage blood flow and prevent stiffness but overdoing it can cause setbacks.

The key is balance, enough activity to aid circulation without putting stress on the surgical site.

Stage 4: Remodeling and Maturation (3 Weeks)

Once the initial healing is well underway, your body shifts its focus toward strengthening and reorganizing the new tissue. At around three weeks, collagen fibers that were rapidly laid down begin restructuring into more organized, stronger patterns. Your scar might still appear red, slightly raised, and sensitive to touch, but improvements should become noticeable.

At this point, gentle scar massage can be initiated. This practice helps align collagen fibers properly and reduces adhesion formation beneath the skin. Light physical activity may begin now with special consideration to avoid working out the areas of trauma. Focus toning activity more on the areas not affected by the trauma while still avoiding cardio activity.

Stage 5: Focused Remodeling (4-6 Weeks)

At the four-week mark, collagen reorganization continues to become more pronounced. The scar tissue gains additional strength and flexibility yet may still appear slightly red or discolored. It is common for itching or tightness to occur during this phase, indicating ongoing tissue remodeling.

Enhanced attention to scar management continues to benefit recovery. Consistent scar massage, maintaining good hydration, and careful sun protection help reduce potential discoloration and promote optimal tissue health. Check with your surgeon to see if topical scar creams like Aquaphor® or topical silicone creams can be applied. They may aid in creating a smoother scar surface. Typically, silicone tape or creams may be applied to the scar starting at week five but not over scabs or open (weeping) areas.

### Stage 6: Consolidation (6-12 Weeks)

By six weeks post-surgery, scar tissue is increasingly stable, with improved strength and flexibility. The redness begins to fade significantly, and your scar may start to feel smoother and less prominent. Nevertheless, continued mild discomfort or sensitivity is normal and part of the healing trajectory.

At this stage, ongoing practices like massage therapy, moisturizing, and diligent sun protection remain crucial. Light to medium physical activity, guided by your healthcare professionals, supports circulation and reduces residual stiffness.

### Stage 7: Established Remodeling (12-16 Weeks)

At twelve weeks, your body has significantly advanced the remodeling process. Your scar is now likely to be flatter, softer, and more closely resembling the surrounding skin tone. Collagen fibers have mostly reorganized into efficient patterns, enhancing the integrity of the healed tissue.

While the scar continues to mature, maintaining consistent skin care practices such as scar tissue therapy, lymphatic drainage massage, moisturizing, and protection from UV rays continues to be important. Continued patience and adherence to these guidelines will ensure the best possible final appearance and function of your healed tissue.

### Stage 8: Intermediate Remodeling (4 to 6 Months)

In this intermediate phase, your body further refines the scar tissue. The collagen continues to align more precisely, increasing the strength and elasticity of the healing tissue. Your scar will continue to lose its redness, becoming paler and less noticeable. However, it's common for the scar to occasionally itch or feel tight as the underlying tissue adjusts and matures.

Consistency remains key during this stage. Ongoing massage therapy not only improves collagen organization but also supports local blood flow and lymphatic drainage, reducing residual swelling and stiffness. Scar tissue therapy is still recommended at this time with sessions being about 3-4 weeks apart. Continued use of sun protection remains critical, as UV exposure can darken scars and impair the remodeling process.

Stage 9: Advanced Maturation (6 to 12 Months)

This final stage marks the completion of scar maturation. At this point, your body fine-tunes the remodeling process, significantly improving the appearance and texture of the scar. Collagen fibers become fully mature, aligning in the most efficient patterns to ensure durability and flexibility. You will notice the scar fading, becoming flatter, softer, and often barely visible.

While improvements become subtler in this advanced stage, continued care ensures the best possible outcome. Scar tissue therapy and moisturizing with topical creams can keep the skin supple and reduce lingering stiffness or discomfort. Patience remains crucial, scar maturation is gradual, and final results often take up to a year or longer. Continued sun protection and avoiding excessive strain on the area remain essential practices to maintain the integrity and aesthetic quality of your healed tissue.

## Differences in Procedure Recovery Times

With all surgeries, getting to the proper recovery specialist as soon as possible is vital. While some surgeons may not allow physical therapy for the first four weeks, other recovery activities, such as post-surgical lymphatic drainage massage, can take place during that time. The body starts throwing down scar tissue as soon as the surgery is completed - you want to make sure you are not giving it too much of a head start or the results will be less than optimal.

Not all surgeries heal equally. Recovery time varies depending on the procedure's complexity, the extent of tissue trauma, and your body's unique physiology. A minimally invasive procedure may allow you to return to normal life within days, while major surgeries may require months of rehabilitation.

## Recovery Highlights - Cosmetic Procedures

Cosmetic procedures often focus on appearance but can involve extensive tissue manipulation:

- **Brazilian Butt Lift (BBL)**: Initial discomfort and positioning restrictions make this a unique recovery. Patients must avoid sitting directly on their buttocks for at least 4-8 weeks and use special pillows or cushions for several weeks beyond that. Swelling may last several weeks, and final contour results can take 3–6 months to appear.
- **Facelift/Neck Lift**: Swelling and bruising peak during the first week. Most patients resume social activities within 4–6 weeks, though full healing can take 3–6 months.
- **Liposuction**: Compression garments are essential for contouring. Bruising typically fades by week four, but results are often not final until month six.
- **Breast Augmentation with Adipose Tissue (Fat)**: Recovery time and outcomes vary based on the surgical technique used. With fat augmentation, swelling and bruising typically subside in a few weeks, and results continue to improve over several months as the body integrates the transferred fat. Proper support through supportive bras and limited upper body activity during early healing is critical to ensure optimal outcomes.
- **Breast Augmentation with Implants over the Muscle:** Implants placed over the muscle cause less

post-operative pain and allow for faster recovery but may result in more visible rippling or shifting. Proper support through supportive bras and limited upper body activity during early healing is critical to ensure optimal outcomes. Recovery often takes eight weeks or longer allowing time for the implant to settle into the tissue pocket.

- **Breast Augmentation with Implants under the Muscle**: Implants placed under the muscle often take longer to settle, up to six months or more, as the muscle gradually stretches and adapts to the implant. Proper support through supportive bras and limited upper body activity during early healing is critical to ensure optimal outcomes.
- **Tummy Tuck**: This procedure has one of the longest recovery timelines, up to a year for complete healing. Most patients return to light activity in 4–6 weeks and continue to recovery for an additional six weeks. Any correction of the diastasis recti (separation of the rectus abdominus muscle) can lengthen the recovery time for healing. Best results are achieved with the use of proper compression for 12-weeks or longer.

## Recovery Highlights – Orthopedic and Trauma Related Surgeries

With reconstructive and trauma related surgeries, these tend to have functional, as well as cosmetic, goals:

- **Knee Replacement**: Physical therapy is vital in restoring function and strength. One often overlooked therapy is the importance of initiating post-surgical manual lymphatic drainage (MLD) within the first 5–10 days post-surgery. Early MLD can help reduce post-surgical swelling, improve joint mobility, and minimize the risk of fibrosis, which can affect long-term outcomes. Patients are encouraged to seek a certified lymphatic therapist familiar with training in orthopedic recovery to optimize this stage of healing. Walking often begins within the first few days, and strengthening exercises are introduced progressively by physical therapists. Despite this rapid initiation of mobility, full recovery, especially return to prior athletic function or long-distance walking, can take up to 12 months.

- **Hip Replacement**: Recovery from hip replacement typically involves fewer initial mobility restrictions compared to knee replacement, but long-term strength and range of motion are equally important. Patients often begin walking with assistance within a few days of surgery. Physical therapy focuses on gait training, balance, and strengthening surrounding muscles. Although pain may subside quickly, regaining full mobility and endurance may take 6 to 12 months. Long-term outcomes are most successful when patients adhere to rehabilitation and engage in regular low-impact physical activity such as swimming or cycling. Again, early post-surgical MLD treatments can help reduce post-surgical swelling, improve mobility, and minimize the risk of fibrosis, which can affect long-term outcomes.
- **C-Sections**: The skin may heal in 6 weeks, but the deeper tissues, especially muscles and fascia, require several months. One highly beneficial, yet often underutilized, therapy during this period is postpartum visceral massage. This form of therapy gently manipulates the abdominal organs and fascia to improve circulation, release adhesions, and promote organ alignment and mobility. Visceral massage can alleviate pelvic congestion, aid digestion, and reduce post-surgical tightness and discomfort in the abdominal region. In addition, general manual lymphatic drainage (MLD) is strongly recommended

for postpartum individuals, especially those who have undergone surgical deliveries. C-sections can lead to swelling not just at the incision site but throughout the body, due to fluid retention and lymphatic system disruption. MLD helps stimulate lymph flow, reduce systemic edema, and relieve the aches and fatigue often reported in the weeks following surgery. Integrating both visceral massage and MLD into the recovery plan can help restore balance and comfort to the body more quickly and effectively.

- **Post-Mastectomy Reconstruction**: Healing varies, influenced by whether radiation or multiple surgeries are involved. Two of the most common reconstruction techniques are implant-based reconstruction and autologous tissue reconstruction, such as the DIEP (Deep Inferior Epigastric Perforator) flap surgery. Both procedures come with physical and emotional adjustments, and patients should receive counseling on what to expect during each phase of healing. Post-operative support garments, scar care, post-operative lymphatic massage, and attention to donor site mobility are all essential for optimal recovery.

Consider scheduling post-op massage therapy sessions sooner rather than later. Even if the therapist cannot work on the surgery area, they can work on areas of the body compensating for the trauma.

Generally, a good rule of thumb is to respect your body's pace. The absence of pain does not always mean full healing, and pushing too soon can cause setbacks.

## Common Misconceptions About Recovery

As mentioned in the introduction, there are many myths claiming effective or fast healing. While some method may work for one person, it doesn't make it applicable to all.

### Myth 1: "Pain Equals Healing"

While some discomfort is expected, persistent or escalating pain is not a badge of honor, it could signal complications like infection or hematoma (Reid et al., 2015). Effective pain management includes both medication and gentle movement, which promotes circulation and healing.

The belief that pain is a necessary indicator of progress may lead patients to ignore warning signs or avoid reporting their symptoms. In truth, unrelenting pain often signals the healing process has gone off course. Infection, internal bleeding, or nerve involvement may present as sharp, throbbing, or radiating pain that increases rather than decreases over time.

Modern recovery protocols emphasize comfort as a priority, recognizing that pain relief can support faster healing. By managing pain effectively, patients are more likely to move, eat, sleep, and breathe deeply, all of which improve oxygenation and tissue repair. Ignoring pain or trying to "tough it out" can result in delays, complications, or even re-hospitalization.

### Myth 2: "Bruising and Swelling Are the Same"

Bruising is the result of blood vessel injury; swelling is caused by fluid and lymph accumulation. They may appear together but are treated differently. Lymphatic drainage massage, ice (when approved), compression, and hydration can reduce swelling, while time and gentle circulation help bruises fade (Atiyeh et al., 2015).

This misconception can lead to confusion when patients try to monitor their healing progress. A large, deep bruise may look alarming but be completely normal, while mild swelling that does not resolve could indicate fluid buildup, a seroma, or lymphatic blockage. Each symptom requires its own approach.

Understanding the difference empowers patients to take proactive measures. Bruises typically change color and fade over days or weeks. Swelling, however, can be managed through elevation, compression garments, and MLD. Persistent or asymmetrical swelling should prompt further evaluation, as it could signal seroma formation or an inflammatory response. Swelling can also be a sign of an allergic reaction, especially if it involves a new medication or new food. For example, Arnica, a popular diuretic herb, can cause allergic reactions in people with hay fever.

Myth 3: "Scarring Is Unavoidable"

Scars are a natural outcome, but their appearance can be minimized with proper care. Silicone-based treatments, scar massage, hydration, and sun protection all contribute to better scar aesthetics (O'Brien & Jones, 2013).

The assumption that scars will always look thick, raised, or discolored can discourage patients from investing in scar care. Consistent and informed aftercare can make a dramatic difference. Research shows that early intervention with silicone sheeting, along with daily massage and moisturizing, can improve both the texture and color of scars.

Sun exposure is one of the biggest culprits in scar discoloration. UV rays can cause scars to darken permanently, especially in the first six months. Patients who protect scars from sunlight, by covering them or using high-SPF sunscreen, often see better long-term cosmetic results. Education and diligence make scar minimization a realistic goal.

Myth 4: "Rest Is the Best Recovery Method"

Too much rest can increase the risk of blood clots and prolong stiffness. Controlled movement, walking, stretching, or prescribed physical therapy, improves circulation and shortens healing time (Mustoe et al., 2002).

Many patients are understandably cautious after surgery and may be afraid that any movement will "undo" their procedure.

However, this fear can lead to stagnation, delayed healing, or secondary complications like pneumonia or deep vein thrombosis (DVT). Movement is not the enemy; it is part of the recovery solution.

Post-operative protocols now encourage early, guided movement tailored to the type of surgery and patient ability. Even gentle activities such as ankle pumps or short walks around the room can stimulate blood flow and oxygenate healing tissues. Activity must be balanced with rest, but complete immobility is rarely beneficial after the first 24–48 hours.

## The Importance of an Individualized Recovery Plan

There is no universal timeline for healing. Your age, medical history, nutrition, hydration, and even stress levels influence recovery speed. That is why individualized recovery plans are essential.

Working closely with your surgeon and post-operative lymphatic massage therapist and, when needed, a rehabilitation team ensures that your plan includes wound care, mobility goals, nutritional strategies, and scar management. Education and support lead to better outcomes.

Recovery is about "getting back to normal" and it is about "moving forward, informed and empowered." If you were active before surgery, you will want to be active after recovery but, like anything else we do, recovery needs to be well-orchestrated based on the surgery or trauma. By understanding the science behind healing, listening to your body, and taking proactive steps, you set the stage for the best possible outcome.

# Chapter 2
## Preparing for Surgery

Preparation is the foundation of a smooth recovery after surgery or any major medical procedure. Research has shown that patients who take an active role in their pre-operative care experience fewer complications, shorter hospital stays, and improved overall outcomes (Albertsmeier et al., 2014). Proper preparation helps optimize immune function, reduces inflammation, and ensures the body is in the best condition to heal efficiently. The better prepared you are before your surgery, the more comfortable and effective your recovery will be.

Imagine preparing for surgery as if you are training for an important athletic event, the better your preparation, the stronger your performance, and the smoother your recovery will be. Studies consistently confirm that patients actively involved in pre-operative care experience fewer complications, shorter hospital stays, and significantly improved outcomes (Albertsmeier et al., 2014). Proper preparation not only primes your body for healing but strengthens your mental resilience, reducing anxiety and enhancing overall recovery.

A structured pre-operative plan can also improve mental resilience, reducing anxiety and post-surgical stress. Prehabilitation, engaging in specific exercises, dietary adjustments, and stress management techniques before surgery, can enhance post-operative healing, particularly in patients undergoing major procedures (Carli et al., 2010). This chapter will guide you through essential steps to take before surgery, including pre-operative health considerations, setting up a recovery-friendly environment, and mental preparation to optimize your experience.

## Optimizing Your Physical Health

The state of your body going into surgery sets the stage for your recovery. Patients who enter surgery in peak health experience significantly faster healing, fewer complications, and better long-term results (Moore et al., 2014). Gentle, regular exercise plays a crucial role. For instance, one notable study found patients who engaged in pre-operative exercise programs had shorter hospital stays and noticeably improved mobility post-surgery (Santa Mina et al., 2014).

Simple, low-impact activities like walking, stretching, and deep breathing exercises can profoundly influence your recovery. These movements enhance circulation, reduce the risk of blood clots, and boost your overall stamina, key factors for quick and complication-free healing (Pedersen & Saltin, 2015).

## Nutrition: Fuel for Healing

Just as athletes fine-tune their diets for optimal performance, what you consume before surgery deeply affects your body's ability to repair itself afterward. Adjust your diet for optimal performance 3-4 weeks prior to surgery. Then when you get closer to the surgery date, be sure to follow any dietary and medication restrictions given to you by your doctor.

Protein stands as the essential building block, vital for collagen production and immune function (Phillips, 2016). Lean proteins such as chicken, fish, eggs, tofu, and legumes will empower your body to efficiently heal incisions, rebuild muscle tissue, and minimize inflammation.

Micronutrients are equally crucial. Vitamins and minerals like vitamin C and zinc accelerate wound closure and strengthen immunity, safeguarding against infection (Carr & Maggini, 2017). Prioritize nutrient-rich foods like citrus fruits, bell peppers, spinach, and nuts to naturally boost your vitamin intake, or supplement with a quality multivitamin when dietary choices are limited.

Interestingly, emerging research highlights the role of gut health in surgical outcomes. Consuming a high-quality probiotic may bolster immune function and reduce inflammation after surgery, enhancing your overall recovery experience (Ouwehand et al., 2002).

Conversely, reducing inflammation-promoting foods can make a remarkable difference in your recovery. High sugar intake has been linked to slower wound healing and increased inflammation, amplifying swelling and discomfort post-surgery (Liu et al., 2014). Cutting back on processed snacks, sugary beverages, and fast food, even briefly, sets a solid foundation for a smoother recovery.

Of course, there may be some foods to avoid the week before, or a couple days before, your surgery, too. Always ask your surgeon if there are any dietary restrictions necessary before you show up for your procedure.

Do not overlook hydration. Drinking at least 8-10 glasses of water daily not only enhances circulation but also prepares your body to better manage anesthesia and reduces post-operative swelling.

## Navigating Medications and Supplements

Medication management before surgery is a delicate balance requiring clear communication with your healthcare providers. Common medications and supplements, including aspirin, ibuprofen, fish oil, and herbal remedies like garlic or ginkgo biloba, can thin blood and heighten the risk of surgical complications (Levine et al., 2014). Consult with your surgeon to pause or adjust medications appropriately to ensure safety and promote optimal healing.

Always discuss these supplements with your medical team to tailor a safe and effective pre-surgical regimen.

## Breaking Bad Habits: Smoking and Alcohol

Smoking cessation and limiting alcohol consumption represent some of the most impactful changes you can make before surgery. Nicotine constricts blood vessels, severely restricting the oxygen and nutrients reaching healing tissues. Studies consistently report significantly higher rates of complications, delayed wound healing, and increased infection rates among smokers (Sorensen, 2012). Ideally, quitting smoking at least 6 weeks before surgery can dramatically improve your outcomes. Your surgery is expensive and spending an additional 3-4 months visiting a wound care specialist to care for tissue necrosis can be burdensome both financially and mentally.

Alcohol similarly affects surgical outcomes by thinning blood, impairing liver function, and exacerbating swelling. Refrain from alcohol intake beginning 4 weeks before surgery. Reducing alcohol intake pre-surgery minimizes these risks, ensuring your body is primed for optimal healing and less prone to complications (Lieber, 2004).

## Building Physical Resilience

Strengthening your body does not require intensive training but rather gentle, consistent effort. Activities like yoga, swimming, or daily walks significantly enhance cardiovascular health and circulation, boosting your body's oxygen delivery and healing potential (Pedersen & Saltin, 2015). For upcoming abdominal procedures specifically, gentle core strengthening exercises like pelvic tilts, leg lifts, and diaphragmatic breathing can improve mobility and reduce post-operative discomfort.

## Setting Up for Success: Creating a Recovery-Friendly Environment

Imagine returning home post-surgery to a comforting, thoughtfully arranged space designed to support your healing. Patients who proactively set up recovery areas report reduced stress, increased comfort, and smoother healing journeys (Levi et al., 2018). Create your "recovery zone" a week or two before your surgery date. Include things that bring you comfort or joy. Supportive pillows, conveniently placed essentials, easy-to-wear clothing, and pre-prepared nutritious meals can drastically reduce unnecessary movement and strain on healing tissues (Gurtner et al., 2011).

What does a recovery zone contain? Consider this checklist:

- **Furniture & Positioning:** Recliner or adjustable bed or wedge to help maintain semi-upright position to reduce swelling and improve breathing.
- **Bedside Table:** with organizer trays to keep medications, snacks, tissues, and remotes within arm's reach.
- **Supportive Pillows:** Wedge, body, or donut pillows to elevate limbs, support your back, or reduce pressure on surgical areas.
- **Lap Desk or Adjustable Tray Table:** Enables comfortable eating, journaling, or using a laptop while resting.
- **Clothing & Comfort:**
    - Loose, easy-to-wear clothing such as front-zip hoodies, button-downs, oversized robes—avoid overhead garments post-surgery.
    - Compression garments or binders (as prescribed): Important for swelling management and tissue support.
    - Non-slip socks or slide-on slippers: Prevents falls and makes short walks safer.

- Hygiene & Wound Care: Antibacterial soap and hand sanitizer to minimize infection risk before handling wounds or drains.
- Moist towelettes and dry shampoo: useful when showering is not possible in early recovery.
- Drain log sheets or app to track post-surgical drain output, if applicable.

- **Nutrition & Hydration:**
    - Pre-prepared, low-sodium meals or meal delivery to reduce the effort of cooking; meals should be protein- and fiber-rich to aid healing and prevent constipation.
    - Electrolyte packets or rehydration drinks (low sodium): Supports hydration, especially if appetite is low or you're on medications.
    - Reusable water bottle with straw: Easy to sip from reclined positions; encourages steady hydration.
- **Medication & Recovery Aids:**
    - Pill organizer or dispenser with timer to help manage pain meds, antibiotics, and supplements on schedule.
    - Cold packs or gel wraps (if approved): For managing pain or localized swelling during the first 72 hours.
- **Post-surgical Supplies:**
    - Gauze, tape, gloves, silicone scar gel, or dressings as recommended by your surgeon.
- **Mental & Emotional Support:**
    - Books, audiobooks, puzzles, or streaming content: Keeps your mind engaged without needing to move.
    - Noise-canceling headphones or calming music to block disruptive sounds, promotes rest.
    - Notebook or recovery journal to track symptoms, mood, progress, and questions for your care team.

- **Support & Communication:**
    - Phone charger with extended cord to keep your phone within reach.
    - List of emergency contacts and surgeon's instructions. Print it and keep it visible near your bed.

## Mental and Emotional Preparation

Psychological readiness is equally crucial for recovery success. Pre-surgical mental preparation reduces anxiety, enhances pain control, and fosters greater satisfaction with results (Moser et al., 2019). Realistically preparing for temporary post-surgical changes like swelling and bruising helps mitigate emotional distress and promotes positivity. Be sure to get your research from reputable sites like National Institute of Health (NIH) or peer-reviewed publications. Remember, information found on Facebook and TikTok is suspect at best. Don't believe everything you find on the Internet.

Techniques like mindfulness meditation and visualization exercises have shown remarkable efficacy in lowering pre-operative anxiety and enhancing post-operative comfort (Zeidan et al., 2011). Establishing a relaxation routine, communicating openly with your surgeon, and connecting with friends and relatives who have undergone similar procedures will further solidify your mental resilience, guiding you toward a smoother, more satisfying recovery.

# Chapter 3
## Traveling for Surgery

With the rise of medical tourism and specialized surgical centers, many patients travel domestically or internationally for surgery and other medical procedures. Traveling for surgery can provide access to top specialists, cost savings, or a more private recovery. However, it requires careful planning. This chapter will guide you through the essential steps of traveling for surgery, from selecting a medical facility to post-surgical care at your home away from home.

Each section will explain why these factors matter, offering deeper insights into making well-informed decisions. Understanding how to navigate safety protocols, recovery environments, and aftercare will empower you to manage potential challenges and achieve the best possible results.

### Researching the Medical Facility and Personnel

Choosing the right medical facility is crucial. A successful outcome depends on the surgeon's skill, the facility's standards, and the quality of post-operative care. Beyond medical competence, the healthcare environment itself significantly impacts recovery.

When evaluating a medical facility, it is essential to consider factors beyond the credentials of the surgeon. Hospitals and clinics that maintain international accreditation standards provide reassurance about their safety, hygiene, and operational protocols. Accredited institutions often undergo regular audits to ensure they meet stringent medical and ethical standards.

Additionally, surgeons who practice at reputable hospitals are more likely to stay up-to-date with the latest surgical techniques and technology, leading to better patient outcomes.

Access to specialized post-operative care is another factor that should not be overlooked. Many top facilities offer integrated care teams which include surgeons, anesthesiologists, and post-operative specialists such as nurses, physical therapists, and manual lymphatic drainage specialists. This comprehensive approach can significantly reduce the risk of complications, particularly for complex procedures requiring longer recovery times.

Furthermore, the medical facility's technological capabilities play a vital role. Advanced medical equipment, including robotic surgical systems and enhanced imaging technologies, can improve precision during procedures. High-quality diagnostic tools are also essential for accurate pre-operative planning and post-operative monitoring.

Another critical aspect is the hospital's emergency response readiness. Complications, though rare, can arise unexpectedly. Facilities with intensive care units (ICUs), well-trained emergency staff, and established medical protocols are better equipped to handle emergencies swiftly and efficiently.

Finally, consider the facility's commitment to patient comfort and well-being. Hospitals or surgery centers offering private rooms, dedicated recovery areas, and patient support services contribute to a more comfortable healing process. Some facilities even provide counseling services and mental health support, acknowledging the emotional and psychological challenges that can accompany surgery.

By carefully selecting a medical facility that excels in these areas, you can maximize your chances of a successful procedure and a smooth recovery. Informed decisions about your medical care ultimately lead to better health outcomes and a more positive surgical experience.

**Why It Matters**

- **Medical Expertise**: A highly experienced surgeon minimizes surgical risks and enhances aesthetic outcomes (Eaves et al., 2013).
- **Accreditation**: Facilities with international accreditations meet high safety and hygiene standards.
- **Emergency Preparedness**: Ensures swift action in case of complications.
- **Post-Operative Care**: Quality aftercare reduces the risk of infection and promotes faster recovery.

**Key Considerations**

- **Verify Credentials and Accreditation**
    - Ensure the surgeon is board-certified by recognized medical boards like the American Board of Plastic Surgery (ABPS).
    - Check for accreditation from organizations like the Joint Commission International (JCI) or Accreditation Association for Ambulatory Health Care (AAAHC).
    - Research online reviews and patient testimonials to gain insights into previous patient experiences.
- **Assess Hospital Safety and Emergency Protocols**
    - Confirm the presence of intensive care units (ICUs) and specialized staff.
    - Inquire about the hospital's infection control protocols (World Health Organization, 2016).
    - Ensure the facility has a contingency plan for medical emergencies.
- **Evaluate Post-Operative Care Services**
    - Availability of lymphatic drainage therapy and wound care specialists can promote proper healing (Földi et al., 2019).
    - Confirm 24/7 medical staff availability for monitoring.

## Pre-Surgery Travel Preparation

Traveling for surgery involves more than booking a flight and securing accommodation. You will feel fine traveling to your destination, but coming home could be challenging. Careful preparation ensures that both the procedure and recovery process are smooth and safe. From navigating legal requirements to addressing the physical and emotional challenges of surgery, thorough planning sets the foundation for a successful experience.

When traveling internationally, understanding the healthcare regulations of the host country is essential. Different regions may have varying standards of care, legal protections for patients, and protocols for addressing medical complications. Familiarizing yourself with these policies can prevent unexpected legal and financial issues.

Financial planning also plays a significant role. Beyond the cost of the procedure itself, consider expenses for travel, accommodations, post-operative care, and unforeseen medical needs. Many medical tourists choose to purchase specialized travel insurance that covers complications, cancellations, or emergency medical evacuations.

Language and cultural differences can present additional challenges. Some hospitals offer translation services and international patient coordinators to facilitate communication between patients and medical staff. Taking advantage of these services ensures clear understanding and informed decision-making throughout your medical journey.

Furthermore, emotional preparation is just as important as logistical planning. Surgery can be physically and mentally demanding, particularly when away from the comforts of home. Having a support system, whether a trusted companion or virtual mental health support, can alleviate anxiety and promote a smoother recovery.

Meticulous planning reduces uncertainty, allowing you to focus on healing and achieving your desired outcome. Each step of preparation, from gathering medical records to coordinating post-operative care, contributes to a more positive and stress-free experience.

**Why It Matters**

- **Health Optimization**: Arriving early allows your body to adjust to new surroundings and possibly a different time zone, reducing surgical risks.
- **Emergency Readiness**: Being prepared with medical documents ensures prompt and accurate treatment if complications arise.
- **Comfort and Convenience**: Thoughtful packing reduces physical strain and facilitates a stress-free recovery.

**Key Considerations**

- **Plan Your Travel Timeline**
    - Arrive 2-3 days early to acclimate, especially when crossing time zones.
    - Allow sufficient recovery time before returning home to minimize risks of blood clots (Kuipers et al., 2011).
- **Pack Thoughtfully**
    - Bring medical records, prescriptions, and consent forms. Consider storing these documents electronically (and encrypted) on a cloud drive in case the paper versions get lost or stolen.
    - Pack comfortable clothing that allows easy dressing post-surgery. Forget vanity – pack for comfort and convenience.
    - Carry necessary medications and check their legal status at your destination. Not all medications (even with a prescription) are allowed to be brought into foreign countries. Of specific concern are cannabis and its derivatives. In addition, over-the-counter drugs purchased overseas may be prohibited in the USA without a doctor's prescription.

    - Prepare electrolyte packets and protein snacks for post-operative nutrition. Remember, non-processed foods are usually prohibited from crossing international borders (meat and plant products).
- **Arrange a Travel Companion**
    - A travel companion can provide essential support for mobility, medication management, and emotional reassurance.

## Where to Stay for Recovery

Post-operative recovery requires an environment conducive to rest and healing. Whether staying in a hotel, rental apartment, or specialized recovery retreat, the right choice can significantly influence the healing process. The recovery period is a critical phase where proper rest, reduced stress, and controlled surroundings contribute to better healing outcomes.

A specialized recovery retreat often provides the most comprehensive post-operative support. Staffed with medical professionals, these retreats offer round-the-clock nursing care, lymphatic drainage therapy, and personalized meal plans tailored to promote healing. Such environments minimize the risk of infection by maintaining stringent cleanliness protocols. Additionally, being surrounded by medical professionals ensures early intervention if complications arise, reducing the need for emergency hospital visits.

Alternatively, staying in a hotel with amenities like room service, adjustable beds, and accessible bathrooms can be beneficial. Some hotels even collaborate with medical facilities to accommodate post-operative patients, providing additional services like in-room nursing care or medication management. Hotels are ideal for those undergoing minor procedures that do not require intensive monitoring.

However, it is important to verify whether the hotel is located near the medical facility for ease of access in case of follow-up appointments or emergencies. Some hotels prohibit post-operative patients for a variety of reasons including wanting to minimize their liability for any emergency situations. It is wise to call ahead.

Rental apartments or private residences provide greater privacy and comfort for longer recovery periods. Patients who prefer a more familiar, homelike environment may benefit from this option, especially if traveling with the family. Having a dedicated caregiver or hiring professional nursing assistance can further enhance the recovery experience. Ensure the space is prepared with necessary supplies, including comfortable bedding, medical supplies, and easily accessible meals.

Moreover, consider noise levels, ventilation, and hygiene standards when selecting accommodations. Noise disturbances can disrupt sleep and slow down recovery, while poor air quality may increase the risk of infection. Properties with elevators and minimal stairs are essential for patients with limited mobility.

The right recovery setting balances comfort, safety, and accessibility. Careful consideration of your medical needs, the level of support available, and proximity to your surgical center will ensure a smoother recovery journey. Prioritizing your healing environment is an investment in your long-term health and well-being.

**Why It Matters**

- **Enhanced Comfort**: Peaceful environments reduce stress and accelerate recovery.
- **Medical Accessibility**: Proximity to healthcare facilities ensures immediate medical assistance if complications arise.
- **Emotional Well-being**: Recovery centers often offer psychological support and companionship, easing the emotional burden of post-surgical recovery.

**Key Considerations**

- **Surgical Recovery Retreats**
  - Offer specialized post-surgical care, including nursing assistance and therapeutic services.

    - Provide controlled environments designed to minimize infection risks.
- **Hotels vs. Short-Term Rentals**
    - Choose accommodations with elevators, room service, and access to medical facilities. Check with the facility for any restrictions.
    - Opt for a location that provides quiet, away from bustling tourist areas.

## Traveling Home After Surgery

The journey home presents unique risks, especially following major surgery. Taking precautions can prevent complications and ensure comfort. After surgery, the body is in a vulnerable state, and external stressors like extended travel times, limited mobility, and pressure changes during flights can exacerbate discomfort and delay healing.

Booking direct flights and requesting assistance at the airport can reduce strain. Have a travel companion to help with luggage, mobility, and emotional support to make the trip smoother and less stressful.

When flying, most aircraft have a pressure altitude of around 8,000 feet. Just like being up in the mountains at 8,000 feet, your body may increase swelling in areas like neck, face, arms and even breasts if not compressed or wrapped. Additionally, the likelihood of developing blood clots, swelling, and deep vein thrombosis (DVT) increases, particularly during long-haul flights. Without proper movement, blood circulation can become sluggish, leading to complications. Preventive measures such as wearing compression socks, performing seated leg exercises, and staying hydrated can mitigate these risks.

Pain management is another crucial factor. Managing post-surgical pain during travel is necessary for comfort and safety. Medications should be taken as prescribed, and having additional pain relief options like cold packs can provide extra comfort.

Furthermore, wound care requires attention during the journey home. Improper handling or significant pressure on the surgical site can lead to infections, swelling, or delayed healing. Dressing supplies, antiseptic wipes, and antibiotics should be readily available.

By planning for these potential challenges, patients can minimize complications, reduce discomfort, and ensure a safer, more comfortable journey back home. A carefully managed travel experience contributes to faster recovery and improved overall outcomes.

**Why It Matters**

- **Blood Clot Prevention**: Extended inactivity during travel increases the risk of deep vein thrombosis (DVT).
- **Wound Management**: Poor handling of wounds can lead to infection.
- **Pain Control**: Adequate pain management ensures a more comfortable journey.

**Key Considerations**

- **Prevent Blood Clots and Swelling**
  - Wear compression socks and compression garments when traveling to enhance circulation.
  - Perform seated leg exercises and walk periodically during long flights (Kuipers et al., 2011).
- **Request Accommodations**
  - Arrange wheelchair assistance at the airport.
  - Book direct flights when possible, to reduce travel time.

## Final Thoughts

Traveling for surgery can be a transformative experience when approached with careful planning and consideration. Not only do you get the surgery you want, but with careful planning, you can have a mini vacation during the days prior.

By selecting accredited facilities, preparing thoroughly, and securing a comfortable recovery environment, you can minimize risks and maximize results. Thoughtful decision-making ensures not only a successful surgical outcome but also a smoother, more comfortable recovery.

In addition to physical recovery, the emotional and psychological aspects of your experience are equally important. Many patients experience feelings of vulnerability, anxiety, or even loneliness during their recovery period. Surrounding yourself with a strong support system, whether through family, friends, or professional counseling, can offer comfort and reassurance.

Furthermore, maintaining open communication with your healthcare provider during your recovery ensures any complications or concerns are addressed promptly. Scheduling virtual follow-ups or telehealth consultations can provide peace of mind and continuity of care. Ask about emergency services after returning home. Should you go to the emergency department if the worst happens such as an infection or the incision opens?

It is also beneficial to monitor your body's signals closely. While minor discomfort and fatigue are typical, persistent, or severe symptoms may indicate a complication requiring medical attention. Keep track of your symptoms, follow all prescribed post-operative instructions, and adhere to your medication regimen to optimize healing.

Financial planning remains an essential consideration even after your surgery. Unexpected medical expenses or additional treatments may arise, so having a contingency budget can reduce stress. Additionally, maintaining thorough medical records can facilitate insurance claims or future follow-ups.

Lastly, remember that recovery is a gradual process. Patience and self-care are key. By taking an active role in your recovery, attending follow-up appointments, and gradually resuming activities, you can achieve the best long-term outcomes.

Traveling for surgery can indeed be a life-enhancing decision, granting you access to specialized care and transformative results. With careful planning and comprehensive post-operative support, you can navigate the challenges of recovery and look forward to a healthier future.

# Chapter 4

## The First 72 Hours

Recovery is just as important as the surgery itself. Whether you have undergone a cosmetic procedure, reconstructive surgery, or orthopedic repair, how you care for your body post-surgery determines how well and quickly you heal. A well-structured recovery plan helps minimize pain, reduce complications, and optimize long-term results. This chapter will guide you through what to expect during the initial days, the first 72 hours. You will learn how to managing pain and discomfort, reducing swelling and bruising, monitoring for complications, and ensure long-term success in healing.

## What to Expect for Recovery

The first three days after surgery are often the most challenging. During this time, your body is in an acute healing phase, working to control bleeding, prevent infection, and begin tissue repair. Swelling and bruising will peak during this period, and discomfort levels will be at their highest. The inflammatory phase of healing is crucial as it sets the foundation for tissue regeneration (Gurtner et al., 2011). While this phase can be difficult, understanding what to expect and how to manage it can ease anxiety and promote a smoother recovery.

These early hours are also critical for emotional adjustment. Many patients are surprised, and sometimes shocked, by how different their body appears immediately after surgery, swollen, bruised, and bandaged. Mentally preparing for this can make a significant difference in emotional resilience.

Support from loved ones or a caregiver can be invaluable during this time, providing comfort and assistance with daily tasks while you focus on healing. Be sure your caregiver is comfortable with seeing you swollen and bruised; not everyone can tolerate seeing or working with bandages and dried blood.

**What to Expect:**

- **Swelling and Bruising:** These will peak within the first two to three days and gradually subside. Prepare yourself for what you may see.
- **Discomfort and Fatigue:** Your body is directing energy toward healing, making rest crucial. Sleep is your body's friend, but so is movement. When you are tired, rest.
- **Drainage or Oozing:** Some procedures involve temporary drains or mild incision leakage. If you cannot stand the sight of your own blood, then ask your companion to help. Drains need to be cared for a few times each day. Bandages need to be changed.
- **Limited Mobility:** Depending on the procedure, mobility may be restricted for a few days. Don't overdo it. Take your time and ask for help.
- **Medication Use:** Pain management and antibiotics are often required. While prescription pain killers are nice and very effective, consider switching to over-the-counter pain medications as soon as possible to minimize constipation, gut issues, and addictions.

## Managing Pain and Discomfort

Medication is the most common method of pain management. Many surgeons prescribe a combination of prescription painkillers and over-the-counter medications, such as acetaminophen or ibuprofen, to balance pain relief with reduced side effects. Multimodal pain management strategies, which combine diverse types of pain relief methods, can reduce opioid dependence and improve recovery outcomes (Buvanendran & Kroin, 2009). Non-medication approaches, including cold therapy, deep breathing, and meditation, can also play a crucial role in keeping discomfort under control (Zeidan et al., 2011).

Incorporating lifestyle strategies alongside medication can make pain management more effective. Creating a calming environment, using aromatherapy, maintaining a structured sleep schedule, and engaging in relaxing music or audiobooks can all help distract from discomfort. These holistic approaches not only ease pain but also promote a sense of control during a time when many aspects of life feel restricted.

**Strategies for Managing Pain**

- **Take Medication as Prescribed:** Follow dosage guidelines and do not skip doses.
- **Use Cold Therapy:** Applying cold packs (if approved) can numb the area and reduce inflammation. Avoid hot packs or heating pads in the first 72-hours unless prescribed by your physician.
- **Incorporate Gentle Movement:** Light stretching or walking can prevent stiffness and improve circulation.
- **Practice Relaxation Techniques:** Deep breathing, meditation, and guided imagery can ease tension and pain perception.
- **Adjust Sleeping Position:** Sleeping with proper support can prevent unnecessary strain on surgical sites.
- **Post-Operative Lymphatic Drainage Massage:** By a well-qualified therapist can help to reduce pain, prevent stiffness, reduce bruising, and decrease swelling.

## Post-Surgical Drains

During the initial 72 hours following surgery, it is common for patients, particularly those undergoing cosmetic or reconstructive procedures, to be discharged with surgical drains in place. These small, flexible tubes are inserted near the incision site to remove excess fluid, such as blood and lymph, which naturally accumulates in the body during the healing process. Drains are essential in preventing complications like seromas (pockets of fluid) or hematomas (collections of blood), which can delay healing, increase infection risk, and distort surgical outcomes (Kim et al., 2015).

There are several types of drains and several sizes, but the most common in post-cosmetic procedures are **closed-suction drains**, such as the Jackson-Pratt (JP) or Blake drains. These function by creating negative pressure to draw fluid out of the surgical site into a small, bulb-shaped reservoir. The reservoir must be emptied and measured regularly, typically every 4-6 hours during the first 72 hours, to monitor output volume and clarity. This information helps the surgical team determine when it is safe to remove the drain, which is usually when daily output falls below a certain threshold, often around 30 mL in 24 hours (Pannucci et al., 2012).

Proper drain care is crucial in reducing infection risk. Hands should always be washed before and after handling the drain, and the insertion site should be cleaned daily as advised by your surgeon. Patients should avoid pulling or kinking the tubing and keep it pinned securely to clothing to prevent accidental dislodgement. If fluid suddenly becomes bright red, foul-smelling, or stops draining altogether, these may be signs of a complication and should be reported immediately to your healthcare provider.

While drains can be uncomfortable, they play a critical role in reducing postoperative swelling and tension on sutures, which helps promote optimal healing and minimizes scarring. Studies have shown that early fluid evacuation via drains contributes to smoother recoveries and may reduce the incidence of surgical site infections in high-risk procedures (Chaudhry et al., 2020). Your surgeon will provide individualized guidance on how long to expect the drains to remain, but most are removed within 3 to 10 days, depending on the volume and nature of the fluid.

When drains are present, patients may still receive post-surgical MLD massage as long as the therapist is familiar with and trained in working around drains. It is very beneficial for the patient to receive post-op MLD sessions with drains in place because lymphatic fluid now has another place to exit the body – through the drains.

## Reducing Swelling and Bruising

Interventions such as lymphatic drainage massage and compression therapy can significantly reduce post-operative swelling and improve patient comfort (Földi et al., 2019). A well-trained post-operative (MLD) massage therapist is an expert in post-op recovery. A massage therapist with basic MLD training is **<u>not</u>** the same as a post-op MLD therapist. Be sure to ask for credentials and training. As a guide, post-op MLD should not be done with creams, lotions, tools, sticks, heat, rollers, or anything other than hands. Also, post-op MLD techniques are always gentle, with some discomfort, but not pain.

What you eat can also help reduce inflammation. Foods and their components, like turmeric (curcumin), arnica, bromelain (found in pineapple), and quercetin (found in kale, red and yellow onions, broccoli, green peppers, tomatoes) can reduce bruising and inflammation in post-surgical patients. The diuretic nature of these foods helps promote urination which is part of the body's cleansing process.

Consistency in managing swelling and bruising is key. Starting with small, manageable steps, like elevating your feet or drinking herbal teas with anti-inflammatory properties, can make a noticeable difference. Minimize sodium on foods and in drinks. Keeping a recovery journal to track changes in swelling and bruising can also help identify what strategies work best for your body and make you feel more engaged in your own healing process. Most often how you feel now is a result of what you ate 5-8 hours ago!

**Tips for Minimizing Swelling and Bruising**

- **Wear Compression Garments:** These help limit fluid retention and support healing tissues.
- **Elevate the Affected Area:** Keeping the surgical site elevated reduces fluid buildup.
- **Stay Hydrated:** Drinking water helps flush excess fluids and toxins from the body.
- **Use Cold Therapy (If Advised):** Applying ice packs intermittently can reduce swelling.
- **Consume Anti-Inflammatory Foods:** Pineapple, turmeric, kale, tomatoes, red or yellow onions, and leafy greens can help decrease inflammation.

## Avoid Incisional Drainage

There is a trend in the post-op recovery community, in some parts of the world, supporting incisional drainage as a post-surgical recovery method. Specifically, some "massage therapists" are opening incision sites after liposuction, tummy tucks, and other cosmetic procedures, and manually squeezing fluid out of the body onto towels, gauze, or whatever happens to be convenient. In many instances, this is being done in hotel rooms, recovery houses, and at home.

Let's be clear. Incisional drainage is not post-operative manual lymphatic drainage (MLD). It is outside the scope of practice (illegal) for massage therapists in the USA to do this. Incisional drainage is a medical procedure which should be done at a doctor's office or medical facility by a licensed medical profession or under medical supervision.

Incisional drainage is a valid post-operative intervention sometimes required when fluid, such as pus from an infection or excess serous fluid, accumulates beneath a surgical incision. This buildup can lead to swelling, discomfort, delayed healing, and even the breakdown of the surgical site if not properly managed. While patients may be tempted to "drain" what appears to be fluid buildup themselves, attempting to express fluid from a healing incision outside of a medical setting can be extremely dangerous.

Improper drainage techniques can introduce new bacteria into the wound, cause tissue trauma, disrupt internal sutures, or mask more serious complications such as abscess formation or deep wound infections (Mangram et al., 1999).

Incision drainage should always be performed under sterile conditions by a healthcare professional who can assess whether the fluid is benign or a sign of infection requiring further treatment such as antibiotics or surgical intervention. Self-treatment can worsen outcomes and significantly delay the healing process while causing the scars to increase in size and shape.

## Monitoring for Complications

Post-surgical infections remain a primary concern. Proper wound care and early detection can reduce infection rates (World Health Organization, 2016). Patients should follow all post-operative care instructions, including keeping incisions clean and dry, taking medications as directed, and attending follow-up appointments. If any concerning symptoms develop, it is crucial to contact a healthcare provider immediately. Infections often present as a new, red, hot to the touch area that can be painful or even oozing. If something like this is found, send a photo to your surgeon or make a trip to the emergency department or urgent care facility.

Blood clots, while unusual, can develop post-operatively, especially for those individuals with certain medical conditions or a family history of blood clots. Any deep vein is susceptible to clot formation, but they usually develop in the leg. Symptoms can include: swelling, pain, tenderness, warmth, and discoloration in the affected leg. Deep vein thrombosis (DVT) prevention strategies, such as early ambulation and compression therapy, significantly lower the risk of post-surgical blood clots (Kuipers et al., 2011).

Beyond physical symptoms, patients should also monitor their emotional and cognitive responses. Confusion, mood swings, or unusual fatigue can sometimes indicate an adverse reaction to medication or an underlying issue such as infection. Documenting symptoms and communicating them with your care team ensures prompt interventions and helps build a safer recovery experience.

**Signs of Potential Complications**

- **Signs of Infection:** Increased redness, warmth, pus, or fever over 100.4°F.
- **Excessive Bleeding:** Persistent bleeding that does not stop with light pressure.
- **Severe Swelling or Pain:** Worsening pain or swelling beyond the expected timeframe.
- **Shortness of Breath or Chest Pain:** May be signs of a blood clot or pulmonary embolism.
- **Wound Dehiscence:** Incision edges pulling apart or excessive fluid leaking from the wound.

## Emotional Stages During Recovery

Surgical recovery is not solely a physical journey, it is also an emotional one. Patients may experience wide ranges of emotions that mirror the psychological stages of trauma recovery. These stages, denial, bargaining, depression, anger, and acceptance, are common psychological responses to significant life events, including medical procedures that alter one's physical appearance or capabilities. Understanding these stages can help patients normalize feelings and seek support if needed (Kubler-Ross & Kessler, 2005).

**Denial**

In the days immediately following surgery, patients may experience denial. This often manifests as emotional numbness, disbelief, or minimization of the surgery's impact.

Denial serves as a protective mechanism, giving the mind time to process the physical and emotional changes occurring. It is not uncommon for patients to express surprise or say, "This doesn't feel real," especially when looking at surgical results for the first time.

**Bargaining**

As reality sets in, some individuals may enter a bargaining phase, where they reflect on hypothetical scenarios like, "If I had prepared better, maybe this wouldn't hurt so much," or "If I follow every instruction perfectly, I'll heal faster than expected." While this stage often involves unrealistic thinking, it can also motivate patients to take recovery seriously. Acknowledging these thoughts and speak with a healthcare professional to help ground expectations.

**Depression**

The depression stage can be particularly challenging. Feelings of regret, sadness, and even hopelessness may arise, especially if the healing process is slower than anticipated or if temporary disfigurement (swelling, bruising, asymmetry) is hard to accept. Research has shown that post-operative depression is not uncommon and may affect up to 20% of patients undergoing elective surgery (Honigman et al., 2004). Support from friends, family, and mental health professionals is crucial during this phase.

**Anger**

Anger and frustration can emerge in response to discomfort, restrictions, or perceived delays in healing. Patients may feel angry at their medical team, their bodies, or even themselves. It is important to recognize anger as a valid response to the disruption that surgery causes. Channeling this energy into constructive actions, such as journaling or engaging in physical therapy, can help release tension in a healthy way.

**Acceptance**

The final stage of emotional recovery is acceptance. Here, patients begin to see their new body or restored function with appreciation and confidence. Scars may still be visible, and discomfort may linger, but the individual begins to feel emotionally at peace with the surgical decision and its outcome. Acceptance is not about loving every part of recovery, it is about acknowledging progress and reclaiming a sense of control and well-being.

Recognizing and respecting each emotional stage during recovery is just as important as adhering to physical post-operative protocols. Whether you are struggling or thriving, your emotional response is valid. Reaching out for emotional support when needed is a vital part of whole-person healing.

## Beyond the 72-Hours

Patients should continue following their surgeon's recommendations well beyond the first 72-hours. Consistent post-operative care, including follow-up visits, adherence to scar treatment protocols, and continued nutritional support, can enhance long-term healing outcomes (Mustoe et al., 2002). Engaging in physical activity, maintaining a nutrient-dense diet, and practicing scar management techniques, such as silicone gel treatments or massage, can ensure that results remain optimal (O'Brien & Jones, 2013). Emotional well-being is also important during this phase, as adjusting to changes in appearance or mobility may take time.

Long-term recovery also presents a valuable opportunity to reflect on the journey and make sustainable lifestyle changes. Many patients find renewed motivation to adopt healthier eating habits, consistent exercise routines, and improved self-care practices. Embracing this transformation not only supports physical healing but can also reinforce emotional satisfaction with your decision to undergo surgery.

Recovering from surgery requires time, patience, and a commitment to post-operative care. By understanding what to expect in the early days, managing pain effectively, minimizing swelling and bruising, monitoring for complications, and maintaining long-term recovery habits, patients can achieve the best possible surgical outcomes. Taking an active role in recovery not only ensures a smoother healing process but also enhances overall well-being and satisfaction with results.

# Chapter 5

## Gender-Affirming Surgery Recovery

All surgeries are traumatic whether deep at the bone or superficial at the skin level. The reason for the surgery does not make the recovery any harder or easier – it is still a difficult and slow process. However, using all available resources to guide your recovery to the best possible outcome will allow your body (and mind) to have the best possible results.

Gender-affirming surgery is a life-changing step for many transgender individuals, offering the opportunity to align physical characteristics with gender identity. These procedures include a range of surgical interventions, such as top surgery (mastectomy for transmasculine patients or breast augmentation for transfeminine patients), bottom surgery (vaginoplasty, phalloplasty, or metoidioplasty), and facial gender-affirming surgeries (such as brow bone reduction, jaw contouring, or tracheal shave). While the emotional and psychological significance of these surgeries is profound, the physical recovery process is equally important and should not be underestimated.

Just like all surgery procedures, each type of gender-affirming surgery carries its own unique recovery demands. However, those demands are not unlike similar surgeries for other reasons. Top surgery, for example, often involves the placement of surgical drains, compression garments, and several weeks of activity restrictions to minimize complications such as fibrosis, seroma or hematoma formation – just like a mastectomy or breast reconstruction. Bottom surgery procedures, particularly vaginoplasty or phalloplasty, require extensive post-operative wound care, catheter management, and possibly regular dilation to maintain neovaginal depth and flexibility. Facial gender-affirming surgeries may result in significant swelling, bruising, and temporary sensory changes, which can take weeks to months to resolve fully just like other face-lift procedures. Your body, in each area, heals the same way irrespective of the reason for the surgery or trauma.

While many patients are highly prepared for the surgical procedures themselves, post-operative recovery protocols are sometimes overlooked or underestimated. The "rules of recovery" do not change just because the surgery is called something different. Recovery for surgery to the face or neck is the same irrespective of the name of the procedure. Likewise, surgery recovery for procedures for the chest are very similar regardless of gender, sex, or procedure. The body really does not care what the procedure is called, it just wants to repair the damage and get back to homeostasis.

One of the most beneficial yet underutilized, and possibly not well known, aspects of post-operative care for transgender surgery patients is post-surgical manual lymphatic drainage (PS-MLD) therapy. PS-MLD is a gentle, non-invasive massage technique designed to stimulate lymphatic flow, reduce swelling, promote healing, and enhance comfort during the early recovery phase. Scar tissue therapy is another recovery tool available as well.

After surgery, lymphatic vessels can become congested or temporarily or permanently disrupted due to inflammation and tissue trauma. This can lead to prolonged swelling (edema), tissue tightness, and discomfort. By gently guiding lymphatic fluid toward functioning lymph nodes, PS-MLD assists the body in removing excess fluid and cellular waste. Research has shown that PS-MLD can accelerate the reduction of post-operative edema, decrease bruising, and support pain relief, making it an ideal adjunct therapy in the early stages of recovery (Lee & Hwang, 2017); (Al Mofeez et al., 2021).

For transgender individuals undergoing extensive tissue manipulation or grafting, as in phalloplasty or vaginoplasty, PS-

MLD can also play a critical role in preventing complications such as fibrosis, which is the formation of dense, fibrous scar tissue. Early and consistent PS-MLD sessions, starting within the first 3-7 days post-op, can support tissue health and flexibility, as well as reduce the risk of fluid pockets that may otherwise require drainage or further medical intervention.

Contributing positively to the emotional aspect of healing, the gentle, structured nature of PS-MLD therapy can offer a sense of care and connection at a time when many patients may feel vulnerable or physically limited. For some transgender patients, the physical touch provided in a therapeutic, respectful, and affirming setting can be both healing and empowering.

While many therapists offer MLD massage, few are trained to work on post-surgical patients. It is important that PS-MLD be performed only by trained professionals familiar with post-surgical recovery, preferably those experienced in gender-affirming procedures. Incorrect techniques or premature treatment can cause discomfort or even interfere with the healing process. Patients should check the credentials of the therapist they are considering. Training for PS-MLD therapists need to be more than a YouTube video or book-learning course. PS-MLD can only be learned with hands-on training. Consider asking your surgical team for referrals to licensed massage therapists who specialize in post-operative care.

Taking recovery seriously not only protects the surgical investment but also honors the emotional and physical journey each patient has undertaken. Gender-affirming surgery is a major medical procedure and deserves the same level of post-operative care, attention, and support as any other reconstructive or cosmetic intervention. By combining surgeon-directed care, self-advocacy, and evidence-based therapies like PS-MLD, transgender patients can optimize healing, reduce complications, and move forward with greater comfort and confidence in their bodies.

# Chapter 6

## Managing Swelling and Bruising

Surgery is a traumatic event to the body. Trauma, whether for cosmetic enhancement, medical necessity, or injury repair, is a significant event that sets your body on a path of healing. While achieving your desired outcome is the goal, the recovery process often comes with temporary side effects like swelling and bruising. These are natural responses as the body repairs itself, sending fluids and inflammatory cells to the site of the procedure and scatters collagen proteins widely. This biological reaction is part of your body's defense mechanism, working to protect and heal the damaged tissues.

While swelling and bruising are, to some degree, unavoidable, understanding how to manage them effectively can improve your comfort and recovery time. Taking proactive steps can minimize these effects, prevent complications, and allow you to resume normal activities sooner. Prolonged or severe swelling and bruising may not only delay healing but also increase the risk of secondary complications, such as infection or poor wound healing. That is why it is essential to implement evidence-based strategies for optimal recovery.

The severity and duration of swelling and bruising can vary depending on factors such as the type of procedure, your age, overall health, and how closely you follow post-operative care instructions. Procedures which involve more extensive tissue manipulation, such as facelifts, tummy tucks, or joint replacements, often result in more pronounced swelling and bruising compared to minor surgeries like appendix or gallbladder removal or C-sections.

In this chapter, we will explore the causes of swelling and

bruising in greater detail, breaking down why these symptoms occur and how they serve as a sign of healing. You will learn the science behind the inflammatory response, the role of the lymphatic system, and how different body areas respond to trauma. By understanding what is happening internally, you will be better equipped to manage your recovery.

We will also cover a comprehensive range of strategies to reduce swelling and bruising, from tried-and-true home remedies like cold compresses and elevation to more advanced therapies like lymphatic drainage massage and compression garments. Nutritional support will also be explored, as specific vitamins and antioxidants can accelerate healing and reduce inflammation.

In addition, recognizing when swelling and bruising indicate a more serious issue is crucial. While most post-operative symptoms are harmless and resolve naturally, excessive, or asymmetric swelling, severe pain, or discoloration may warrant immediate medical attention. We will discuss the key warning signs to watch for and how to stay in close communication with your healthcare provider throughout your recovery.

Whether you are recovering from plastic surgery, orthopedic procedures, or even dental work, these practical tips will support your body's healing journey and help you feel your best as quickly as possible. Knowledge is one of the most powerful tools you have in the healing process, and with the right approach, you can navigate your recovery with confidence and ease.

## Swelling and Bruising: Why Do They Happen?

After surgery, your body enters full-on repair mode. **Swelling (edema)** and **bruising (ecchymosis)** are part of the healing process:

- **Swelling** occurs as your body sends extra fluid and white blood cells to the surgical site to aid tissue repair. Surgical procedures often disrupt and destroy lymphatic vessels, which play a crucial role in fluid drainage. When these vessels are damaged, lymphatic fluid can accumulate in the tissues, leading to prolonged swelling and discomfort. The fluid buildup creates puffiness and tenderness, and in some cases, may require targeted therapies such as lymphatic drainage massage to support recovery. When looking at your body in the mirror, most often the swelling you see is free lymphatic fluid between tissue fibers and *not* contained in the lymphatic vessels.

- **Bruising** happens when tiny blood vessels (capillaries) are damaged during surgery, causing blood to leak under the skin and form visible discoloration.

## Types of Bruising

Bruising is not a one-size-fits-all phenomenon. It can vary in severity, depth, and healing time. The main types include:

1. **Petechiae** – Tiny red, purple, or brown spots that result from small capillary bleeds. These often appear after procedures involving delicate areas like the eyes or lips.
2. **Ecchymosis** – The classic bruise, appearing as large patches of discoloration due to blood pooling under the skin. Common after many procedures like facelifts, liposuction, or tummy tucks.
3. **Purpura** – A more severe form of bruising where larger patches of pooled blood do not blanch when pressed. This may indicate underlying coagulation issues.
4. **Hematoma** – Unlike a regular bruise, a hematoma is a collection of blood that forms a firm lump under the skin. While small hematomas resolve on their own, larger ones may require other treatments like cold laser therapy or medical drainage.

5. **Hemosiderin Staining** – Not necessarily a bruise, but it looks like one. Typically found outside the surgery area (like inside of the knee when someone has a tummy-tuck). This is a brownish discoloration of the skin which occurs when the red blood cells break down and leak iron under the skin. The colored area has no pain and may becomes mottled as it heals and disappears on its own.

The severity of swelling and bruising depends on the type of procedure, individual healing response, and how well post-op instructions are followed. Most patients experience peak swelling within 48-72 hours post-surgery, with gradual improvement over the next two to four weeks. Bruising can last 7-21 days, shifting in color as it heals.

## Best Strategies to Reduce Swelling and Bruising

**Compression Therapy**

Compression garments play a key role in post-operative recovery by reducing swelling, improving circulation, and providing structural support to healing tissues. Depending on the type of surgery, different compression methods may be recommended:

- **Wraps & Bandages**: Elastic wraps help control swelling and provide localized pressure to specific areas. Elastic wraps can be used for upper and lower extremities, chin and neck, and the torso. Be careful with wraps as they are easy to overtighten and provide too much compression, starving the tissue of vital fluid exchange.
- **Fajas**: Commonly used after liposuction and abdominoplasty, fajas (compression garment) provide firm compression to sculpt and support healing tissues.
- **Binders**: Used after tummy tucks or abdominal procedures, binders stabilize the midsection and prevent excessive swelling. Binders are a large (9-12 inches wide) elastic wrap.

- **Sleeves & Compression Socks**: These help prevent fluid accumulation in the arms and legs, particularly after surgeries affecting the limbs. Both are available for part or all of the extremity.

Patients should follow their surgeon's guidance on when and how long to wear compression garments, as improper use can affect healing outcomes. However, because many surgeons may not stay up to date on advancements in compression adjuncts, patients should also consult with their lymphatic decongestive therapist for additional guidance on optimal compression use. In most cases, expect to compress for 4-8 weeks or longer, depending on the procedure.

**MEAT or PEACE & LOVE**

Recent research suggests that **MEAT (Movement, Exercise, Analgesics, Treatment)** is more effective as a recovery protocol than the traditional R.I.C.E. method for injury and recovery management (Bleakley et al., 2012). But we all like acronyms, so if a shorter one is good, a longer one must be better, right?

More recently fitness and coaching classes are beginning to promote the **PEACE & LOVE (Protection, Elevation, Avoid anti-inflammatories, Compression, Education & Load, Optimism, Vascularization, Exercise)** framework as presented in the British Journal of Sports Medicine (Dubois & Esculier, 2020). Both emphasize similar recovery principles, one is just more detailed than the other. Both focus on an active recovery instead of excessive immobilization.

**M.E.A.T.**

- **Movement:** Light movement, such as walking or gentle stretching, promotes circulation and prevents excessive fluid retention.
- **Exercise:** Gentle, surgeon-approved exercises can reduce stiffness and speed up lymphatic drainage.
- **Analgesics:** Use cold compresses and pain medications as prescribed to control swelling.

- **Treatment:** Techniques such as lymphatic drainage massage, compression, physical therapy, and proper wound care help optimize healing.

**P.E.A.C.E. (First 1-3 Days)**

- **Protect:** Limit movement or activity which increases pain or threatens the healing tissue. Avoid overloading or returning to full activity too soon, especially in the early inflammatory phase.
- **Elevate:** Raise the injured or operated area above the level of the heart. Promotes fluid drainage through gravity, which can reduce swelling and discomfort.
- **Avoid Anti-inflammatories:** Avoid NSAIDs like ibuprofen in the early stages unless specifically prescribed. Inflammation is a necessary part of healing. Early suppression can delay tissue repair (Gulick et al., 2020).
- **Compress:** Use compression garments, wraps, or bandaging as recommended by your provider. Helps limit swelling, improve proprioception, and stabilize healing tissue.
- **Educate:** Understand your healing process and engage actively in your recovery plan. Empowered patients who understand their condition make better recovery decisions and reduce over-reliance on passive therapies.

**L.O.V.E. (After Acute Phase)**

- **Load:** Reintroduce gentle, progressive movement and resistance under clinical guidance. Encourages collagen alignment, tissue repair, and restores strength/function. Overprotection delays recovery.
- **Optimism:** Psychological well-being plays a key role in healing. Positive mindset, resilience, and reduced catastrophizing improve pain outcomes and functional results.

- **Vascularization:** Engage in pain-free aerobic activity to increase blood flow and oxygen delivery. Walking, cycling, or light swimming supports tissue oxygenation and reduces pain sensitivity. This is also where MLD would be great to aid in the healing process.
- **Exercise:** Prescribed, condition-specific rehab exercise aids return to function. Restores mobility, coordination, and prevents chronic stiffness or deconditioning.

**Post-Surgical Lymphatic Drainage Massage**

Post-surgical manual lymphatic drainage massage is a specialized technique that helps reduce swelling by stimulating the lymphatic system. A systematic review by Földi et al. (2019) confirmed its benefits in reducing post-surgical edema and improving fluid mobilization (Földi, M. et al., 2019).

Lymphatic drainage massage works by gently manipulating the skin in rhythmic motions to stimulate the flow of lymph fluid. Unlike traditional massage, which primarily targets muscles, PS-MLD focuses on the lymphatic vessels just beneath the skin. This encourages the removal of excess fluid and metabolic waste products, which is essential after surgery when the lymphatic system may be overwhelmed or compromised.

Just to be clear, post-op manual lymphatic drainage massage is a more advanced MLD treatment and usually starts from day three post-op. PS-MLD should be performed only by a well-trained Complete Decongestive Therapist (CDT) or PS-MLD therapist since much of your lymphatic system has been compromised during the surgery. Therapists with CDT or PS-MLD training have received four times the training as basic MLD therapists.

Many basic MLD therapists believe they have the knowledge and techniques to work on post-operative clients, but the coursework we have reviewed does not support that claim. Basic MLD therapists should avoid post-surgical clients until at least week seven or eight post-op, once the body is no longer compromised.

PS-MLD massage can accelerate recovery by reducing pain and inflammation. It enhances circulation, delivering oxygen and nutrients to the healing tissues while simultaneously aiding in the removal of toxins and cellular debris. This can be particularly beneficial for patients recovering from liposuction, facelifts, or abdominoplasty, where fluid retention is common. By reducing swelling, PS-MLD also helps surgical results become visible sooner, providing patients with a clearer view of their outcomes.

However, timing is essential. While PS-MLD is safe and effective, using improper techniques can lead to complications. Most surgeons recommend beginning PS-MLD within the first week after surgery. Certified PS-MLD massage therapists are trained to adapt their techniques based on the specific type of surgery performed and the patient's recovery progress.

Furthermore, research supports the psychological benefits of PS-MLD. Gentle, hands-on therapy can reduce anxiety, promote relaxation, and provide comfort during the stressful recovery period. The reduction in discomfort and the visible improvement in swelling can boost confidence and improve overall patient satisfaction.

By incorporating lymphatic drainage massage into their post-operative care plan, patients can enjoy a smoother recovery with reduced swelling, less discomfort, and faster results.

**Stay Hydrated**

Drinking plenty of water (at least 8-10 glasses a day) helps to flush metabolic waste, reduces fluid retention, and keeps circulation moving. A study by Lang et al. (2017) supports adequate hydration in post-surgical recovery, demonstrating improved wound healing in well-hydrated patients.

Water supports the transport of essential nutrients to tissues. When cells receive sufficient hydration, collagen production increases, leading to faster wound closure and reduced scarring. Furthermore, staying hydrated reduces the risk of blood clots, a common post-surgical complication. Proper fluid balance prevents blood from thickening, which lowers the risk of deep vein thrombosis (DVT) and other circulation-related issues.

Within the first 72-hours post-op, electrolyte-rich fluids like coconut water or electrolyte drinks can further enhance hydration by replenishing minerals lost during surgery. However, not all beverages are beneficial. Beverages high in sugar and sodium can increase inflammation, slowing the healing process.

To ensure optimal hydration, monitor your fluid intake and look for signs of dehydration such as dizziness, fatigue, or dry skin. Incorporating hydrating foods like cucumbers, oranges, and watermelon into your diet can provide additional fluids and essential nutrients. By prioritizing hydration, you can support your body's natural recovery mechanisms and accelerate the healing process.

**Adjust Your Diet for Faster Healing**

What you eat plays a significant role in swelling and bruising. Nutrient-rich foods can accelerate the healing process by reducing inflammation, supporting tissue repair, and providing essential vitamins and minerals. On the other hand, poor dietary choices can contribute to increased swelling, prolonged bruising, and slower recovery. Being mindful of your food intake can enhance your body's natural healing response. Some foods actively combat inflammation, while others may worsen it, making dietary management an important aspect of post-surgical care.

*Best Foods to Reduce Swelling and Bruising*

- **Pineapple & Papaya**: These tropical fruits contain bromelain, a powerful enzyme that has been clinically proven to reduce bruising and swelling (Brien et al., 2004). Bromelain has anti-inflammatory and analgesic properties, making it a natural choice for post-operative recovery. Studies show that consuming bromelain supplements or fresh pineapple and papaya can accelerate the breakdown of blood clots and reduce the severity of bruising.

- **Citrus Fruits**: Oranges, grapefruits, lemons, and limes are excellent sources of vitamin C, which is essential for collagen production and tissue repair (Carr & Maggini, 2017). Vitamin C also acts as an antioxidant, protecting cells from damage caused by inflammation. Consuming fresh citrus juice or incorporating these fruits into your diet can strengthen your immune response and support faster healing.
- **Leafy Greens**: Kale, spinach, and Swiss chard are rich in vitamin K, which plays a critical role in blood clotting and bruise healing (Booth et al., 2003). Vitamin K also supports vascular health, reducing the likelihood of excessive bleeding and bruising. Adding leafy greens to salads, smoothies, or steamed meals ensures you receive an ample supply of this essential nutrient. Temper your Vitamin K intake if you are on blood thinners or are at risk of blood clots. Check with your physician.
- **Protein Sources**: Lean proteins like chicken, fish, eggs, tofu, and legumes provide the building blocks your body needs for tissue repair and collagen synthesis (Phillips, 2016). Protein also helps maintain muscle strength during recovery, preventing muscle loss that can occur during periods of inactivity. Aim to include a source of high-quality protein with every meal to support faster healing.
- **Turmeric, Ginger, Red or Yellow Onions, Green Peppers, Tomatoes**: All are renowned for their potent anti-inflammatory properties. Curcumin, the active compound in turmeric, has been shown to reduce inflammation and alleviate pain in numerous clinical trials (Daily et al., 2016). Ginger contains gingerol, which has antioxidant effects and can help manage

post-operative discomfort. Red or yellow onions, green peppers, and tomatoes have quercetin, a flavonoid with anti-inflammatory and antioxidant properties. Consuming turmeric tea, ginger shots, or adding these veggies to meals can aid recovery.

*Foods to Avoid*

- **Sports Drinks**: While electrolyte drinks may seem like a good choice after surgery, many are high in sodium and sugar, which can contribute to fluid retention and prolonged swelling. After the first few days post-op, switch to plain water or coconut water to stay hydrated without the added sodium.
- **Salty & Processed Foods**: High-sodium foods such as canned soups, processed meats, and packaged snacks can lead to increased water retention, worsening swelling. Excess sodium also strains the kidneys, which can slow down the body's ability to regulate fluids. Choose whole, minimally processed foods to avoid these effects.
- **Alcohol & Caffeine**: Alcohol is dehydrating and can interfere with your body's ability to heal (Lieber, 2004). It also dilates blood vessels, potentially worsening bruising. Caffeine, in large amounts, can have similar effects by reducing hydration. It is best to limit or avoid both during the early stages of recovery.
- **Sugary Foods**: Refined sugar is known to increase inflammation and suppress immune function (Liu et al., 2014). Avoid sweets, pastries, and sugary drinks during recovery. Instead, satisfy your sweet tooth with naturally sweet fruits like berries, which offer antioxidants that support healing.

By making mindful dietary choices, you can significantly reduce swelling and bruising, accelerate healing, and improve overall recovery outcomes. Combine proper nutrition with other recommended recovery strategies for the best results.

## The Takeaway

By following these research-backed recovery strategies, controlled movement, proper nutrition, hydration, and lymphatic drainage, you can heal faster and get back to feeling like yourself again. Give your body time, and soon you will be enjoying the results of your transformation.

# Chapter 7

## Wound Care and Scar Management

Surgery is an investment in yourself, and proper wound care is essential to ensure smooth healing and minimize scarring. While your surgeon provides post-operative instructions, understanding how to clean and protect incisions, choose the best scar treatment methods, and recognize warning signs of complications will empower you in your recovery. In this chapter, we will guide you through the best evidence-based wound care and scar prevention practices to help you heal optimally and confidently.

### Understanding the Wound Healing Process

Proper post-operative wound care can significantly impact the long-term aesthetic and functional outcome of scars (Mustoe et al., 2002).

Surgical wounds heal in phases, and each stage requires proper care to reduce complications and optimize recovery:

1. **Hemostasis (Immediate Post-Surgery):** Blood clotting begins immediately to stop bleeding and create a protective barrier.
2. **Inflammatory Phase (1–5 Days Post-Surgery):** White blood cells flood the area to fight infection, and swelling, redness, and mild discomfort are normal.
3. **Proliferative Phase (5–21 Days Post-Surgery):** New tissue forms, and collagen begins repairing the incision site.
4. **Maturation Phase (3 Weeks to 12 Months):** The scar strengthens and gradually fades, becoming less noticeable over time.

Proper wound care during these phases is critical to preventing infection, reducing inflammation, and ensuring optimal healing.

## How to Clean and Protect Incisions

**1. Follow Your Surgeon's Instructions**

- **Your surgeon's post-operative care plan:** It is tailored to your specific procedure, so it is important to adhere to their recommendations regarding wound care, dressings, and activity restrictions.
- **Topicals:** Before applying any topical to an incision, get clearance from your surgeon.

**2. Keep the Incision Clean**

- **Use a gentle, antimicrobial soap**: Once cleared by your surgeon, clean the incision with lukewarm water and a mild, fragrance-free soap. Using a soap with a moisturizing lotion component can help keep your body moisturized while you recover.
- **Pat, do not rub**: Use a clean, soft towel to gently pat the area dry. Even if you still have sutures, be gentle with the wound.
- **Avoid soaking**: Do not submerge the incision in bathtubs, pools, or hot tubs until cleared by your doctor. Submersion is typically not allowed until after all scabbing has disappeared.
- **Let scabs fall off naturally**: Picking at scabs can reopen the wound, cause infection, and increase scarring risk.

**3. Apply Appropriate Dressings**

- **Sterile gauze or surgical dressings**: Your surgeon may give you some guidance on this, but opinions vary. Some surgeons may prefer uncovered incisions while others send you home from surgery with a clear plastic adhesive covering over the incision that stays on for a week or 10-days. The bottom line is all wounds need to be kept clean, free from body oils, dirt, and other components which may cause infection. Any wound can be covered with a breathable, sterile gauze dressing held in place with first-aid tape or post-surgical tape.

- **Hydrocolloid dressings**: Hydrocolloids are moisture-retentive dressings. While that may sound like an optimal environment for wound healing, in most cases, hydrocolloids are not necessary in the early stages of recovery. They are used in some cases for extremely dry scars or wounds going through recovery because of necrosis and debridement. The most popular hydrocolloid dressing is silicone tape or sheets, most often used starting at week 5 post-op.

**4. Prevent Infection**

- **Watch for signs of infection from the inside**: Infection of an incision or scar can occur from the outside or inside. If the surgical area was contaminated with bacteria or other pathogens, infections can occur from the inside. Symptoms of this would be redness and warmth of the skin, tenderness in the area, and possibly oozing from under the skin, pus, increased pain, or fever above 100.4°F. These infections are serious and need immediate attention from your doctor. They will most often prescribe antibiotics to start.
- **Watch for signs of infection on the incision**: Infection of an incision or scar occurs when the incision area is not kept clean. Symptoms may include redness and warmth of the area, tenderness, possibly oozing from the incision, pus, increased pain, or fever above 100.4°F. Any infection is serious and you should consult with your doctor immediately so they can prescribe antibacterial ointment or medicine.

- **Use antibiotic ointments with caution**: Some wounds heal better with minimal topical applications; always follow your surgeon's advice. Don't use over-the-counter triple antibacterial ointment on your wounds and incisions unless you clear it with your surgeon. Neomycin is one of the most common causes of allergic contact dermatitis which presents as an itchy, red rash.
- **Avoid friction from clothing**: Friction can irritate incisions and slow healing. Ensure you are wearing clean clothes each day. Was you faja's and abdominal binders frequently as they tend to get body oils and blood on them from incisions.

## Best Scar Treatment Methods

Scarring is a natural part of healing, but proper care can significantly minimize its appearance. Here are the best evidence-based scar treatments:

**1. Silicone-Based Products**

- **Silicone Tape & Scar Gels**: Many of the silicone tapes and sheets are made from silicone or have one side with a silicone component. Best practice is to use these after all scabs have disappeared. Studies show that silicone helps hydrate the skin, reduce collagen overproduction, and soften scars (O'Brien & Jones, 2013).
- **When to start**: Usually 4-6 weeks post-op.
- **How long to use**: 8–36 weeks for optimal results.

**2. Sun Protection**

- **UV rays darken scars**: Sun screen is going to be a necessary topical on scars for the rest of your life. Scars lack melanin, the pigment in the skin which protects us from the sun's harmful rays. Scars can sunburn and often do. Use broad-spectrum sunscreen (SPF 30 or higher) on healing incisions starting around week six.

- **Cover scars with clothing**: Physical protection is the best way to prevent hyperpigmentation and sunburns on scars and incisions.

**3. Massage Therapy for Scar Remodeling**

- **Gentle scar massage** is a technique used to manipulate the incision while it is healing. Proper technique can break down excess collagen and improve flexibility (Tan & Liu, 2018). Be sure to ask your PS-MLD therapists if they have received hands-on training for scar work. If not, gentle myofascial therapy on the scar will help.
- **Start five weeks post-op** and continue for several months. Be sure the therapist you see has successfully completed training in post-op scar tissue work.

**4. Hydration and Nutrition**

- **Hydrated skin heals better**: Drink plenty of water and use a fragrance-free moisturizer on surrounding skin. Unless cleared by your surgeon, do not apply topicals on the incision.
- **Eat foods with collagen-boosting nutrients**: Vitamin C, zinc, and protein-rich foods aid in tissue repair and scar improvement. Eat a healthy diet to provide your body with all the healing nutrients necessary.

**5. Professional Scar Treatments**

- **Medical Treatments:** For stubborn scars, medical treatments may be beneficial. These treatments are usually performed months after surgery, when your body decides to go a little rogue with scar development:
- **Laser Therapy**: Reduces discoloration and smooths scar tissue.
- **Microneedling**: Stimulates collagen remodeling for improved skin texture.

- **Corticosteroid Injections**: Steroid shots are one of the ways doctors help flatten raised or hypertrophic scars (Manuskiatti & Fitzpatrick, 2022).
- **Surgical Scar Revision**: Reserved for severe scarring that does not improve with conservative treatments.

## When to Seek Medical Help

While most wounds heal without complications, certain symptoms require immediate medical attention. You should be looking at your incision and scar at least daily for anything out of the ordinary. Seek help if you experience:

- **Signs of Infection:** Increasing redness, warmth, pus, fever, or excessive pain.
- **Cellulitis:** A bacterial skin infection that presents with spreading redness, warmth, swelling, tenderness, and sometimes fever or chills. Left untreated, it can progress to more serious complications.
- **MRSA (Methicillin-Resistant Staphylococcus Aureus):** A type of staph infection resistant to many antibiotics. Signs include painful, red, swollen skin lesions that may produce pus or drainage. MRSA infections require urgent medical evaluation and treatment.
- **Wound Dehiscence:** This occurs when a surgical incision reopens either partially or completely due to poor wound healing, excessive tension, or infection. It can lead to serious complications, including exposure of underlying tissues. If dehiscence occurs, seek medical attention immediately to prevent infection and further tissue damage.
- **Excessive Swelling or Fluid Accumulation:** This may indicate a seroma or hematoma.
    - **Seroma:** A seroma is a collection of clear fluid that builds up under the skin after surgery, often at the surgical site. It can cause swelling and discomfort

but usually resolves on its own. In some cases, medical drainage may be necessary.

    - **Hematoma:** A hematoma is a localized collection of blood outside the blood vessels, typically caused by surgical trauma or excessive bleeding. Unlike a seroma, a hematoma can cause significant bruising, firmness, and pain and may require drainage or medical intervention if severe.

- **Unusual Pain Beyond Expected Recovery:** Pain that worsens instead of improving may signal a problem.

## Signs of Pulling a Suture or Excessive Tension

Excessive tension on an incision can lead to more prominent scar development. When an incision is pulled or a suture is pulled, that creates a tear in the tissue which causes the healing process to start over in that immediate area. Here's how you may know if you "pulled a stitch:"

- Sudden sharp pain around the incision site
- Increased redness or swelling
- Small gaps or widening of the wound
- Spotting of blood on dressings

Patients experiencing these symptoms should reduce movement in the affected area and consult their surgeon to prevent further complications.

## The Takeaway

Proper wound care is crucial for minimizing complications and ensuring beautiful, long-lasting surgical results. By following your surgeon's guidelines, keeping your incision clean, using proven scar treatments, and recognizing warning signs, you can optimize your healing process. Remember, scar healing takes time, and patience is key.

# Chapter 8
## Nutrition for Optimal Healing

Proper nutrition plays a vital role in post-surgical recovery. The body requires an increased intake of essential nutrients to rebuild tissues, reduce inflammation, and support immune function. A well-balanced diet can significantly shorten recovery time, reduce complications, and enhance overall healing outcomes (Evans et al., 2020). Proper nutrition can also support the prevention of post-surgical infections and complications such as delayed wound healing and excessive inflammation (de Luis et al., 2021).

In addition to physical benefits, nutrition influences mental health during recovery. Deficiencies in key nutrients can lead to increased fatigue, brain fog, and even depressive symptoms after surgery (Jacka et al., 2017). Nutritional strategies designed to optimize healing can improve both physiological and psychological recovery outcomes. This chapter outlines the best post-surgery diet plan, the most effective vitamins and supplements for healing, and the foods that should be included or avoided in the recovery process.

## Best Post-Surgery Diet Plan

As the body's energy demands increase significantly after surgery, recovery requires additional calories, proteins, and micronutrients to fuel tissue repair and immune defense. A carefully structured diet can accelerate healing and minimize inflammation. The type of surgery may also determine specific dietary needs, with major procedures such as abdominoplasty or orthopedic surgeries requiring higher protein and caloric intake than minor cosmetic procedures (Weimann et al., 2017). Let's look at some of the more important parts of a recovery diet.

**Macronutrient Balance for Recovery**

- **Protein:** One of our body's major building blocks, protein is essential for tissue repair and wound healing. Increasing protein intake post-surgery can enhance collagen synthesis, a key component of skin and muscle regeneration (Børsheim et al., 2008). High-quality protein sources such as eggs, lean meats, fish, and plant-based proteins like lentils and quinoa can significantly improve healing rates. By consuming adequate protein, it may be possible to reduce the risk of post-operative infections (Cereda et al., 2017).
- **Healthy Fats:** We have all heard about healthy fats and unhealthy fats so consider eating food rich in omega-3 fatty acids. You can get these from sources like salmon, flaxseeds, and walnuts. Omega-3 fatty acids help reduce inflammation and support cell membrane integrity (Calder, 2013). You can go one step further and eat foods rich in monounsaturated fats. Consider foods such as olive oil and avocados to improve immune function and cardiovascular health, also crucial for overall recovery.
- **Complex Carbohydrates:** Skip the white bread, sugar, and bananas and go for more complex carbohydrates like whole grains, legumes, and vegetables. These foods take longer to digest and provide sustained energy, prevent post-operative fatigue, and stabilize blood sugar levels. Unlike refined carbohydrates (sugars), whole foods, like granola, supply fiber that supports gut health and prevents digestive issues such as constipation which is often caused by pain medications (Slavin, 2013).

**Hydration, Electrolytes, and Digestion**

- **Water:** Hydration supports circulation, prevents constipation from pain medications plus facilitates nutrient transport. Drinking plenty of water can help all body systems do better. Dehydration leads to increased pain perception and slower tissue regeneration (Popkin et al., 2010). Don't like plain water? Consider adding in a sugar-free flavor additive or simply some lemon juice to make it a little more palatable.

- **Electrolytes:** Minerals like potassium (found in bananas and sweet potatoes) and magnesium (from leafy greens and nuts) help maintain fluid balance and muscle function. Post-operative patients who experience excessive fluid loss or imbalances should prioritize electrolyte-rich foods and supplements (Lobo et al., 2006). Be careful, though, most electrolyte drinks have excessive sodium which will cause more swelling. Consider using the electrolyte drink as a flavor additive to regular water with a 5:1 ratio – split the one bottle of electrolyte beverage across five 24-oz bottles of water.

## Meal Planning for the First Weeks

What does post-surgical meal planning look like and what foods are best to eat? It depends on the surgery, of course. Head and neck surgery may have different requirements than ankle surgery. However, planning an appropriate balanced, highly nutritional meal for each day will get your recovery off to a good start.

- **First Few Days:** Start by eating soft, easily digestible foods like smoothies, yogurts, eggs, oatmeal, soups, and mashed vegetables. These are all easily prepared, easy to eat, and avoid strain on the digestive system. Limit dairy intake and vegetables like cabbage and broccoli that cause gas. This will avoid post-surgical bloating.
- **5-14 Days Post-Op:** Gradually introduce lean proteins (with minimal salt), healthy fats like avocados, and fiber-rich foods like oatmeal and vegetables to support gut health. These foods will also continue to reduce any

constipation, ensuring a smooth and low-effort bowel movement. Incorporating additional low sodium, probiotic-rich foods such as yogurt or kimchi can further improve digestion.

- **Weeks Two to Four:** A fully balanced diet with a variety of whole foods ensures continuous healing and energy replenishment. Patients should continue to prioritize hydration, limit excess salt, increase fiber intake, and avoiding processed foods to reduced inflammation levels and sodium intake.

## Vitamins and Supplements to Speed Recovery

Certain vitamins and minerals play a critical role in tissue regeneration, immune support, and inflammation control. Many post-surgical complications, including poor wound healing and increased infection risk, are linked to nutritional deficiencies (Cereda et al., 2017). Smoking and alcohol consumption should also be avoided throughout the recovery period.

**Essential Vitamins for Healing**

Vitamins are essential for many of our body's functions including repairing tissues after traumas. Many of us do not get proper amounts of all essential vitamins simply through the food we eat. A quality, daily, supplemental vitamin can go a long way to help the body heal.

Vitamins A, C and D are very important for healing. Consider adding these to your diet two-three weeks before surgery so your body is ready to heal after the procedure. Post-surgery, include these in your diet as soon as your appetite returns.

- **Vitamin A:** Essential for epithelial cell repair and immune function. Vitamin A can be found in carrots, sweet potatoes, and dark leafy greens (Stephenson et al., 2020). Deficiencies in vitamin A have been linked to slower wound closure and increased risk of infection.

- **Vitamin C:** A powerful antioxidant that promotes collagen production and strengthens the immune system. Nutritionists have mixed opinions on Vitamin C and the dose necessary for good health. We suggest not using mega-doses of supplements rather, eat the foods high in Vitamin C – most of which are significant contributors to your daily fiber intake. Foods high in Vitamin C include citrus fruits, bell peppers, and strawberries (Carr & Maggini, 2017).
- **Vitamin D:** Supports bone health and immune regulation. Vitamin D is one of the few vitamins we can receive just by sitting in the sun so why not enjoy the relaxation time? Other than the sun, you can get vitamin D from salmon and tuna, eggs, beef liver, and enriched dairy products like yogurts and milk. (Pludowski et al., 2013). Vitamin D deficiency is associated with higher inflammation levels and longer hospital stays following surgery.

**Key Minerals for Recovery**

Our body required certain minerals to rebuild after surgery and trauma. Consider this list as some of the more essential minerals. Talk to your surgeon a couple weeks prior to surgery to see which minerals you should be consuming before surgery and which are better during your recovery. In some cases, certain minerals can complicate the surgical procedure and need to be avoided days before or after surgery.

- **Zinc:** Essential for wound healing, immune regulation, and cellular repair; deficiency can impair tissue regeneration and increase the risk of infection (Lin P.-H. et al., 2017). Foods rich in zinc are many, yet oysters and beef seem to be the highest per serving. Other foods rich in zinc include shellfish, seeds, wheat germ, oats, and nuts. Zinc supplementation may be necessary for individuals with compromised immune systems.

- **Iron:** Supports oxygen transport in the blood, preventing fatigue and enhancing recovery (Beard, 2001). Iron intake requirements differ between males and females and not everyone requires iron supplementation. Foods rich in iron include red meats, poultry, seafood, and eggs. For plant-based iron, consider eating legumes (beans), tofu, and dark leafy greens. Fortified cereals are also a good source of iron. Whichever source you choose, consider a side of foods rich in vitamin C to enhance absorption of the iron.
- **Magnesium:** Helps with muscle relaxation, nerve function, and inflammation control (Rosanoff et al., 2016). Magnesium does not get the recognition it deserves in our diet and magnesium rich foods are often side dishes. Magnesium helps muscles relax and promotes sleep while helping our bodies maintain proper levels of calcium, potassium, and zinc. Yet, most multivitamin supplements contain little magnesium. Foods rich in magnesium include soy products (tofu, soy milk), legumes, seed and nuts, peanut butter, dried apricots, and whole grain products. Patients recovering from musculoskeletal surgeries or experiencing muscle spasms should ensure adequate magnesium intake. Typically the go-to supplement is magnesium glycinate.

**Supplements for Special Cases**

- **Bromelain:** An enzyme in pineapple known to reduce swelling and bruising. It has natural anti-inflammatory and pain-relieving properties, making it beneficial for patients recovering from cosmetic surgeries with significant tissue trauma or hematoma formation (Brien et al., 2004). Do your body good – eat the pineapple rather than drink the juice, and increase your fiber intake at the same time.
- **Collagen Peptides:** May support skin and connective tissue healing. Collagen is a structural protein essential

for wound repair, making it particularly helpful for patients recovering from cosmetic or orthopedic procedures requiring extensive tissue regeneration (Kim et al., 2018).

- **Omega-3 Fish Oil:** Reduces post-surgical inflammation and supports immune function. It is especially useful for individuals undergoing major surgery or those with chronic inflammatory conditions, as it has been shown to lower pro-inflammatory markers and enhance overall recovery (Calder, 2013).

## Summary of Foods to Eat and Avoid

**Healing-Boosting Foods**

- **Lean Proteins:** Chicken, fish, eggs, and tofu support tissue repair.
- **Healthy Fats:** Avocados, olive oil, and nuts reduce inflammation and aid cell growth.
- **Antioxidant-Rich Fruits and Vegetables:** Berries, citrus fruits, spinach, and broccoli enhance immune function.
- **Whole Grains and Fiber:** Quinoa, oatmeal, brown rice, and legumes help digestion and energy levels.

**Foods to Avoid**

- **Processed Foods:** Lunch meat, canned sauces and soups, bacon and ham, high in additives and preservatives which can increase inflammation.
- **Refined Sugars:** Sugar, sweets, syrups, white bread, bananas all may promote inflammation and impair immune function (Lustig, R. H. et al, 2012).
- **High-Sodium Foods and Fast Food:** Yes, french-fries, deli sandwiches, fried burgers, etc. encourage water retention with high sodium.
- **Alcohol and Caffeine:** Dehydrate the body and interfere with medication metabolism.

# Chapter 9

## The Role of Herbs in Post-Surgical Recovery

Recovering from surgery is a complex process involving the management of pain, inflammation, infection prevention, and tissue regeneration. Conventional medical care is still the backbone of post-surgical recovery, but herbal remedies have increasingly gained recognition for their complementary benefits to speedy recovery. Herbs have been used medicinally for thousands of years, across numerous cultures, for their ability to reduce inflammation, alleviate pain, prevent infection, and enhance wound healing. This chapter provides an extensive exploration of the most effective herbs supported by scientific evidence to optimize post-surgical recovery.

It is known that certain herbs may complicate surgical procedures by reducing blood clotting abilities or by causing anesthesia effects to linger longer afterwards. Most often surgeons will advise cessation of garlic, St. John's Wort, Ginkgo, Ginseng, Echinacea, Tocopherol, Ginger, Kava, Ephedra, Fish oil, Valerian, Feverfew, CoQ10, and Dong quai for at least two weeks pre-op.

Please consult your surgeon to discuss which spices and herbs you need to avoid pre-surgery and within the first few days post-surgery.

## Herbs for Inflammation and Pain Management

### Turmeric (Curcuma longa)

Turmeric, containing the powerful compound curcumin, has been extensively studied for its anti-inflammatory properties. Curcumin functions by inhibiting key inflammatory pathways, significantly reducing post-operative swelling and discomfort. Clinical trials highlight curcumin's efficacy, comparing favorably to conventional anti-inflammatory medications (Hewlings & Kalman, 2017). One study found that black pepper enhanced the absorption of turmeric in the body by up to 300%.

**Ginger (Zingiber officinale)**
Ginger contains gingerols and shogaols, compounds with potent anti-inflammatory and analgesic effects. Studies demonstrate ginger's capability in reducing inflammation and pain intensity, particularly beneficial in managing post-operative muscle and joint discomfort (Rondanelli et al., 2020).

**Arnica Gel (Arnica montana)**
Arnica gel (topical) is widely recognized for reducing bruising, swelling, and pain associated with surgical procedures. Topical application of arnica gel directly to the affected area helps minimize inflammation and accelerates the resolution of bruising. Clinical research indicates that regular and early application of arnica gel post-surgery significantly improves outcomes in terms of pain relief, reduction in swelling, and overall tissue recovery. It is crucial, however, to follow precise usage instructions and to avoid applying arnica gel to open wounds or broken skin to prevent irritation or allergic reactions (Iannitti et al., 2016).

**Arnica Tea (Arnica montana)**
Arnica tea, typically used internally in diluted and highly controlled amounts, has traditional roots in herbal medicine for reducing inflammation and internal bruising. While historically valued for internal healing, modern clinical evidence supporting the internal consumption of arnica tea remains limited, and safety concerns due to its potential toxicity must be taken seriously. If considering arnica tea,

consultation with a qualified herbal practitioner or healthcare provider is necessary to ensure safe consumption, appropriate dosing, and to prevent adverse effects. People who are pregnant, breast feeding, or have hay fever allergies should avoid ingesting Arnica Tea.

**Boswellia (Boswellia serrata)**
Boswellia, or Indian frankincense, contains boswellic acids known to suppress inflammatory enzymes. Clinical studies indicate its effectiveness in decreasing inflammation and pain, potentially reducing reliance on conventional painkillers during recovery (Ammon, 2016).

## Herbs to Accelerate Wound Healing

**Aloe Vera (Aloe barbadensis)**
Renowned for accelerating wound healing, aloe vera gel promotes faster tissue regeneration through increased collagen synthesis and reduced inflammation. Clinical evaluations confirm aloe vera's beneficial role in post-surgical wound management and reducing healing time (Hashemi et al., 2015).

**Calendula (Calendula officinalis)**
Calendula possesses remarkable wound healing, anti-inflammatory, and antimicrobial properties. Studies demonstrate that topical calendula significantly enhances collagen production, epithelialization, and reduces healing duration (Preethi & Kuttan, 2009).

**Gotu Kola (Centella asiatica)**
Gotu kola effectively promotes wound repair and improves blood circulation around surgical sites. Clinical trials reveal significant improvements in wound tensile strength, reduced scar formation, and accelerated wound closure following topical application (Brinkhaus et al., 2000).

**Dragon's Blood (Croton lechleri)**
Traditionally used in wound care, Dragon's Blood resin enhances tissue regeneration and prevents microbial infections. Scientific research corroborates its effectiveness in expediting wound healing and reducing bacterial contamination (Porras-Reyes et al., 1993).

## Herbs for Infection Prevention

**Honey**
Honey is a well-documented antimicrobial agent effective against a variety of bacteria. Clinical studies indicate honey's utility in significantly reducing infection rates and promoting a sterile healing environment, especially valuable in surgical wound care (Molan, 2001).

**Tea Tree Oil (Melaleuca alternifolia)**
Tea tree oil exhibits potent antimicrobial properties, valuable in preventing wound infections. Research validates its broad-spectrum effectiveness against pathogens commonly implicated in post-operative infections. Proper dilution and topical application remain essential to avoid skin irritation (Carson et al., 2006).

**Echinacea (Echinacea purpurea)**
Echinacea is recognized for its immune-boosting and antimicrobial properties. Clinical findings suggest echinacea supplementation can enhance immune function, thereby decreasing susceptibility to post-operative infections (Barnes et al., 2005).

**Garlic (Allium sativum)**
Garlic has robust antimicrobial properties due to its active compound allicin. Studies indicate garlic's efficacy in combating bacterial infections, supporting its use as a preventive measure in post-operative care (Ankri & Mirelman, 1999).

## Additional Herbs for Comprehensive Recovery

**Lavender (Lavandula angustifolia)**
Lavender oil, known for its calming and analgesic properties, aids relaxation and reduces anxiety associated with surgical recovery. Aromatherapy with lavender significantly decreases stress hormones and promotes better sleep quality, essential for effective healing (Malcolm & Tallian, 2017).

**Chamomile (Matricaria chamomilla)**
Chamomile provides soothing anti-inflammatory and calming effects beneficial for reducing stress, anxiety, and inflammation during the post-operative period. Clinical evidence supports chamomile's role in enhancing overall patient comfort and accelerating recovery processes (Amsterdam et al., 2009).

## Safety and Precautions

While herbal remedies offer numerous benefits, safety and correct usage are paramount. Interactions between herbs and conventional medications must be carefully considered, and consultation with healthcare providers is essential prior to incorporating herbal supplements into recovery protocols.

## Conclusion

Herbs present a valuable complementary approach to conventional post-surgical care, providing natural solutions for pain management, inflammation control, wound healing acceleration, and infection prevention. With proper integration and medical oversight, herbal remedies can significantly enhance surgical outcomes and patient satisfaction.

# Chapter 10

Post-Surgical Bodily Functions

Post-surgical recovery extends far beyond incision care and managing pain. In the weeks following surgery, many patients experience temporary, but sometimes distressing, changes to fundamental bodily functions. These include constipation, urinary frequency or retention, changes to the menstrual cycle, digestive disruptions, vaginal issues, sexual difficulties, impotence, and nausea or vomiting. While most of these complications resolve naturally with time, understanding them can reduce anxiety, prevent complications, and support smoother healing.

This comprehensive chapter explores some of these common post-operative issues, drawing from current medical research, clinical recommendations, and patient experiences. It provides practical strategies for managing symptoms, knowing when to seek help, and returning to normal function safely.

## Constipation After Surgery

Constipation is one of the most common early post-operative concerns. Studies report up to 60% of patients experience difficulty with bowel movements in the first week post-surgery (Bharucha et al., 2013). Always an unpleasant experience, care for constipation is necessary to avoid other issues days later. If left unaddressed, severe constipation can lead to discomfort, bloating, and in extreme cases, complications such as bowel obstruction.

**Why It Happens**

Multiple factors contribute to post-operative constipation:

- **Anesthesia and Medications:** General anesthesia slows down bowel motility, and opioid painkillers further inhibit digestion.
- **Immobility:** Reduces peristalsis, the natural movement of the digestive tract.
- **Low Fiber Intake:** Immediately after surgery, many patients consume a soft or liquid diet, which may lack sufficient fiber to promote regular bowel movements.
- **Dehydration:** Proper hydration is necessary for digestion and stool formation. Without adequate fluid intake, stools become harder and more difficult to pass.

**Prevention and Treatment**

- **Hydration:** 2–3 liters per day, unless medically restricted (Popkin et al., 2010).
- **Increase Fiber Intake:** Consider increasing your overall fiber intake a month before surgery. Whole grains, oatmeal, legumes, fruits, and vegetables are rich in fiber, which adds bulk to stool and promotes movement through the intestines (Slavin, 2013).
- **Use Natural Laxatives:** Foods like prunes, chia seeds, flaxseeds, and psyllium husk have natural laxative properties that can gently stimulate bowel movements (Lever et al., 2019).
- **Pharmacologic Interventions:** Stool softeners (docusate), osmotic laxatives (MiraLAX), or stimulants (senna). Magnesium citrate (ingredient in Milk of Magnesia) may also help.
- **Abdominal Massage:** May support peristalsis, the movement of matter through the colon.
- **Incorporate Probiotics:** Fermented foods such as yogurt, kefir, and sauerkraut introduce beneficial gut bacteria that aid digestion (Ouwehand et al., 2002).

- **Encourage Gentle Movement:** Walking and light stretching can stimulate digestion and promote bowel regularity. This is one reason why movement after surgery is preferred over just resting.

## Handling Menstrual Cycle and Disruptions

For women, surgical stress can cause temporary disruption of the hypothalamic-pituitary-ovarian axis, leading to irregular or missed periods (Practice Committee of the ASRM, 2015). In some cases, you may miss your period completely for up to six weeks. In other instances, your cervix may spot for a couple of weeks post-op. It varies greatly depending on your body, your age, and how the trauma of surgery affects you.

**Pads vs. Tampons**

During post-surgical recovery, especially in the first few weeks after procedures involving the abdomen, pelvis, or genital region, most healthcare providers recommend using external menstrual hygiene products like pads rather than internal options such as tampons or cups. Tampons can increase the risk of introducing bacteria to healing tissues and may disrupt the delicate balance of the vaginal microbiome, potentially leading to infection or delayed healing, especially when surgical drains or incisions are nearby.

Additionally, inserting tampons or cups may cause strain or discomfort if abdominal or pelvic muscles are healing from surgery. Pads, while less discreet, offer a safer, non-invasive option that minimizes the risk of contamination or pressure on healing tissues. Patients are typically advised to wait at least 4-6 weeks or until cleared by their surgeon before resuming tampon use after surgery (American College of Obstetricians and Gynecologists [ACOG], 2020).

Of course, if your surgery was a breast lift or even liposuction, something not within the abdominal cavity or pelvic floor, then the choice of pad, tampon, or cup is a personal preference. If you are unsure, please consult with your medical care team.

**Menstrual Cup**

Menstrual cups can be a convenient and eco-friendly alternative to pads or tampons, but their use immediately after surgery, particularly abdominal, pelvic, or cosmetic procedures such as tummy tucks or labiaplasty, should be approached with caution. During the post-operative healing phase, especially within the first few weeks, inserting or removing a menstrual cup may place unnecessary strain on internal or external sutures, increase intra-abdominal pressure, or introduce bacteria to healing tissues.

While there is limited direct research on menstrual cup use post-surgery, general surgical guidelines recommend avoiding internal menstrual products until cleared by a healthcare provider, particularly in surgeries involving the pelvic floor or reproductive system (North, Oldham, & Gannon, 2020). Patients should consult their surgeon before resuming menstrual cup use to ensure it won't interfere with healing, drain placement, or incision integrity.

**What to Expect with Your Menstrual Cycle**

- **Delayed Ovulation:** Stress and inflammation may suppress the hormonal cascade.
- **Missed or Spotty Periods:** Especially common after general anesthesia.
- **Heavier or Lighter Bleeding:** Changes in clotting or uterine responsiveness.

**Management**

- **Cycle Tracking:** Use apps or journals to note changes.
- **Nutrition and Iron:** To support hormonal and red blood cell recovery.
- **Medical Review:** Seek medical consultation if your changes persist longer than three cycles.

## Urinary Issues

Urinary function is often impacted by anesthesia, medications, catheter use, and pelvic floor strain. In most surgeries, you can expect a catheter to be used. There may be a little tenderness for a day or two post-op while urinating. If you have blood in the urine or sharp pain while urinating, consult with your surgeon or post-op nurse. Urinary tract infections happen in both male and female patients, treat them right away.

**Types of Dysfunction**

- **Retention:** Difficulty initiating urination or fully emptying the bladder.
- **Incontinence:** Especially after pelvic surgeries due to weakened sphincters.
- **Urinary Frequency:** Often caused by bladder irritation or infection.

Post-operative urinary retention occurs in up to 25% of major surgical patients (Fowler et al., 2008). Catheter-associated urinary tract infections (CAUTIs) occur in 8–15% of cases with prolonged catheterization (Nicolle, 2014).

**Interventions**

- **Timed Voiding:** Urinate every 2–4 hours even without urge.
- **Pelvic Floor Exercises:** Particularly important after gynecological procedures.
- **Hydration and Cranberry Juice:** May help reduce infection risk.
- **Medical Help:** Cloudy, odorous urine, burning, or fever requires testing.

## Digestive Disruptions

Beyond constipation, surgery can trigger gas, bloating, reflux, or indigestion. These symptoms can stem from anesthesia, antibiotic use, stress, and altered gut flora. For the first day or two post-op, consider fluids with carbs and electrolytes. Slowly introduce your digestive system to bland, easy-to-digest foods.

**Common Complaints**

- **Gas and Bloating:** Often caused by slowed motility or antibiotics.
- **Reflux or Heartburn:** Due to increased intra-abdominal pressure or medication.
- **Loss of Appetite:** Often from nausea, taste changes, or emotional factors.

**Nutritional Tips**

- **Eat Slowly:** Helps prevent swallowing air and promotes digestion.
- **Smaller, Frequent Meals:** Easier to digest and maintain energy.
- **Fermented Foods:** Eat yogurt, kefir, kimchi for probiotics (Ouwehand et al., 2002).
- **Avoid:** Carbonated drinks, fried foods, dairy (if sensitive).

## Nausea and Vomiting

Post-operative nausea and vomiting (PONV) affects 20–30% of patients and is triggered by anesthesia, pain meds, and early movement (Apfel et al., 2012).

**Contributing Factors**

- Female gender
- Motion sickness history
- Opioid use
- Laparoscopic or abdominal procedures

**Prevention and Treatment**

- **Antiemetics:** Ondansetron (Zofran), promethazine.
- **Aromatherapy:** Peppermint oil and isopropyl alcohol pads.

- **Herbal Support:** Ginger, chamomile, and lemon balm teas (Ernst & Pittler, 2000).
- **Gradual Diet Advancement:** Clear fluids, then a BRAT diet (bananas, rice, applesauce, toast).

## Sexual Activity and Intimacy

Resuming sexual activity after surgery can be physically and emotionally complex. For most surgical procedures, sexual activity should be avoided for at least a couple of weeks. Movement, pain medication, bruising, and lack of energy will most likely be the deterrents. Give your body a break and let it heal during this time. As you recover, your desire may increase. Supportive communication and gradual reintroduction are key to restoring intimacy (Basson et al., 2010).

**Common Concerns**

- Pain with penetration (especially after pelvic surgery)
- Fear of tearing or damaging surgical sites
- Reduced lubrication from medications or hormone shifts
- Emotional detachment or loss of libido
- Erectile dysfunction

**When to Resume**

- **Non-Invasive Surgeries:** Typically 2–3 weeks with clearance from your physician
- **Pelvic/Abdominal Procedures:** 4–6 weeks minimum, or as advised by your physician

**Supportive Tips**

- Use water-based lubricant
- Try positions that avoid pressure on the surgical area
- Start with manual stimulation, caressing, fondling
- Communicate about comfort, fear, and expectations
- Avoid taking erectile enhancement drugs

## Vaginal Health After Surgery

Hormonal changes, stress, and antibiotics can disrupt the vaginal microbiome. These changes are common and treatable but should not be ignored.

**Possible Symptoms**

- Dryness
- Odor or discharge
- Itching or discomfort
- Recurrent yeast or bacterial infections

**Restoring Balance**

- **pH-Friendly Hygiene:** Avoid douching or fragranced products.
- **Cotton Underwear:** Reduces moisture and irritation.
- **Topical Moisturizers:** Vitamin E suppositories, aloe-based gels.
- **Probiotics:** Lactobacillus supplements or fermented foods (Reid et al., 2001).

**When to Seek Help**

- Symptoms lasting longer than 7–10 days
- Discharge with foul smell, fever, or severe discomfort

## Conclusion

Understanding the body's responses in the first few weeks after surgery can reduce anxiety and promote faster healing. Changes to urination, bowel habits, sexual function, and digestion are all part of the complex recovery process. These transitions are typically temporary, but require attention, patience, and sometimes medical support. Open communication with your provider and self-advocacy are vital for returning to full function and restoring confidence in your body.

# Chapter 11

## Movement & Physical Activity

Movement and physical activity play a pivotal role in post-surgical recovery. From improving circulation and reducing swelling to preserving muscle tone and supporting mental health, the right kind of movement at the right time can significantly impact outcomes. However, determining when and how to resume physical activity requires individualized guidance based on the type of surgery, the extent of trauma, and the patient's overall health.

This chapter explores evidence-based recommendations for post-operative movement by surgery type, outlines week-by-week guidelines for safe activity, addresses when patients can safely return to normal routines, and includes considerations for special populations and emotional well-being.

### How Soon Can You Exercise?

Each type of surgery affects the body differently. Resuming physical activity too early can increase the risk of complications such as wound dehiscence, seroma, and delayed healing. Conversely, avoiding all movement for too long can increase the risk of deep vein thrombosis (DVT), joint stiffness, and muscle atrophy.

In almost all cases, simple walking and movement to get in and out of a chair or bed is allowed from the first day or two. If you plan to take a journey outside, consider taking someone with you for your safety.

When determining if a particular exercise is appropriate during recovery, patients should consider the area of the body affected by surgery. For instance, a patient who has undergone a knee replacement may need to avoid weight-bearing leg exercises early on but can safely perform upper body resistance exercises like bicep curls while seated. Similarly, someone recovering from abdominal surgery may find walking and arm exercises more tolerable than core-focused movements. The key is to select activities that do not strain the surgical site, interfere with wound healing, or provoke discomfort. If in doubt, consulting with a physical therapist or surgeon ensures safety and appropriateness.

**1. Cosmetic Surgery (Lipo, Tummy Tuck, Breast Aug)**

- **First 1–2 Weeks:** Walking is encouraged within 24 hours to prevent blood clots. Avoid lifting, bending, or twisting. According to Matarasso et al. (2014), early ambulation after abdominoplasty reduces the risk of thromboembolic events without compromising healing. In other words, start movement early and reduce your risk of blood clots.
- **Weeks 3–4:** Gentle stretching and longer walks are safe. Avoid core work, upper-body resistance, and impact exercises.
- **Weeks 5–6:** Light strength training and low-impact cardio may resume with clearance.

**2. Orthopedic Surgery (Joint Replacement, ACL Repair, Fracture Fixation)**

- **First 1–2 Weeks:** Passive range-of-motion exercises and guided physical therapy.
- **Weeks 3–6:** Progression to weight-bearing and active range of motion with supervision. Shelbourne and Nitz (2012) found that early movement after ACL reconstruction improved outcomes compared to delayed mobilization.
- **Weeks 6–12:** Return to resistance training, walking, and low-impact cardio.

**3. Gynecological Surgery (Hysterectomy, C-section)**

- **First 1–2 Weeks:** Gentle walking, pelvic floor relaxation, and diaphragmatic breathing.
- **Weeks 3–5:** Light stretching, posture work, and pelvic floor reactivation. Hilde et al. (2016) recommend early pelvic floor engagement to restore continence and support healing after gynecologic surgery.
- **Weeks 6–8:** Gradual return to core and resistance work under supervision.

**4. Cancer/Reconstructive Surgery**

- **First 1–2 Weeks:** Walking, gentle range of motion. Courneya and Friedenreich (2007) emphasize the importance of gradual reconditioning to manage fatigue and muscle loss after cancer treatment.
- **Weeks 3–6:** Lymph drainage movements, posture correction, breathing exercises.
- **Weeks 6–12:** Resistance training and cardiovascular activity under medical guidance.

**5. Abdominal and Hernia Repair Surgeries**

- **First 1–2 Weeks:** Minimal core engagement; prioritize walking and deep breathing.
- **Weeks 3–6:** Gentle stretching, avoid lifting or coughing without support.
- **Weeks 6–12:** Return to core work cautiously with medical clearance.

## Safe Stretches and Gentle Movements (Week-by-Week Guide)

**Week 1**

- **Focus:** Circulation, breathing, preventing stiffness.
- **Movements:**
    - Ankle pumps and toe wiggles
    - Diaphragmatic breathing
    - Shoulder rolls (if permitted)
    - Short indoor walks every 2–3 hours

**Research:** Early ambulation reduces the risk of pulmonary complications and DVT (AORN Guidelines, 2020).

**Week 2**

- **Focus:** Light mobility, maintaining joint function. In addition to Week 1 movements, add in the movements listed here.
- **Movements:**
    - Seated marches
    - Neck and shoulder circles
    - Standing side-to-side weight shifts
    - Wall-supported calf stretches

**Week 3–4**

- **Focus:** Gentle strength and posture awareness. Walking should be at least 1-2 miles a day.
- **Movements:**
    - Standing leg lifts
    - Wall sits (if cleared)
    - Gentle spinal rotations (seated)
    - Pelvic tilts and bridges (non-core surgeries only)

**Research:** Posture exercises after breast surgery reduce postural imbalances and shoulder pain (McNeely et al., 2010).

**Week 5–6**

- **Focus:** Endurance and reactivation. Consider walking at least 2 miles each day, more if you are up for it.
- **Movements:**
    - Light resistance bands (arms and legs)
    - Stationary bike (low resistance)
    - Step-ups
    - Arm circles and gentle yoga stretches

**Week 7–8 and Beyond**

- **Focus:** Functional movement, increased activity.
- **Movements:**
    - Low-impact cardio (elliptical, swimming)

- Pilates and balance exercises
- Resistance training for all major muscle groups
- Longer walks or hikes

**Special Note:** Always avoid movements that cause pain, pulling at incision sites, or dizziness. Progress slowly and consult a professional for individualized guidance.

## Understanding the Body's Pain Signals

Understanding the body's pain signals is an important part of navigating physical recovery. Not all discomfort means the same thing, and learning to differentiate types of pain can help patients make smarter choices about movement. The following table outlines common types of post-operative pain, what they may indicate, and recommended actions patients can take in response.

| Type of Pain | Possible Cause | Recommended Action |
|---|---|---|
| Sharp or Pinching Pain | May suggest nerve irritation or impingement, especially if it radiates. | Stop activity; consult a healthcare provider if it persists. |
| Pulling Sensation | Could indicate premature stretching of healing tissues or tight scar tissue. | Ease up on movement; consult a scar tissue therapist; stretch gently if permitted by provider. |

| Type of Pain | Possible Cause | Recommended Action |
|---|---|---|
| Dull, Deep Ache | Often reflects muscular fatigue; common during reconditioning. | Monitor closely; okay if mild and short-lived. |
| Persistent Aching | May indicate inflammation or overuse. | Rest and reassess activity level; consider modifying routine. |
| Stabbing Pain with Swelling/Redness | Could signal infection or serious post-op complication. | Stop immediately; seek medical attention. |

## When to Resume Normal Activities

Returning to daily activities varies depending on the type of procedure and healing rate. Below is a general guide with common timelines and safety considerations:

| Activity | Typical Timeline | Notes |
|---|---|---|
| Walking up stairs | 1–2 weeks | With support as needed |
| Driving | 2–3 weeks | Must be off narcotics, able to brake safely |
| Desk work | 2–4 weeks | Depends on fatigue and sitting tolerance |
| Lifting groceries | 3–5 weeks | Avoid heavy loads over 10–15 lbs. initially |
| Sexual activity | 4–6 weeks | Wait for wound healing and comfort |

| Activity | Typical Timeline | Notes |
|---|---|---|
| Yardwork or house chores | 5–8 weeks | Avoid repetitive strain until fully healed |
| Jogging or strength training | 6–8+ weeks | Start gradually with medical clearance |

## Special Populations and Considerations

**Older Adults**

- May require longer healing timelines due to reduced muscle mass and joint flexibility.
- Balance exercises and fall prevention are key.

**Obese Patients**

- Risk for wound complications and DVT is higher; walking and water-based movement is encouraged.
- Use supportive garments to minimize tissue strain.

**Immunocompromised Individuals**

- Require more cautious pacing.
- Avoid group settings or gyms to prevent infections.

**Athletes and Active Individuals**

- May experience mental health dips due to activity restriction.
- Gradual progression with rehab professionals reduces injury risk.

## Emotional and Mental Health Benefits of Movement

Early movement during recovery reduces symptoms of anxiety, depression, and post-surgical fatigue (Brosseau et al., 2004). Patients who resume gentle physical activity tend to report:

- Better sleep quality
- Increased confidence

- Lower perceived pain levels
- Improved mood
- Quicker return to normal activities

## Summary and Recommendations

Exercise is always challenging when the body is recovering. Best advice is to start slow and build up your capabilities gradually. Start by walking within 24 hours unless contraindicated, advance slowly with a focus on breath, posture, gait, and circulation. Avoid high-impact or resistance activity until cleared. No running or jumping, please. Get clinical post-op manual lymphatic drainage and scar tissue therapy as soon as possible post-op to help ease movements. Consider using physical therapy when available since they will customize the recovery for your age, body type, and pre-existing conditions. Most of all, don't be discouraged by your limitations – after all, you are in recovery mode.

# Chapter 12

## Lymphatic Drainage and Clinical Massage Therapy

Effective post-operative care goes beyond incisions and bandages. One of the most overlooked but critical elements of recovery is managing the lymphatic and soft tissue systems. Swelling, fibrosis, seromas, restricted movement, and prolonged healing times can often be linked to inadequate attention to these systems. Manual therapies, including lymphatic drainage and clinical massage, offer substantial support for post-operative recovery.

This chapter explores the role of lymphatic drainage and clinical manual soft tissue therapy in surgical healing. Through an understanding of lymphatic function, effective reduction techniques, and the science behind clinical massage therapy, patients and caregivers can optimize recovery outcomes and avoid complications.

Scar tissue work as part of post-operative manual lymphatic drainage sessions will be discussed in another chapter.

### Why Post-Op Lymphatic Drainage Is Essential

The lymphatic system plays a crucial role in immune defense and fluid balance. It consists of a network of vessels and nodes that drain interstitial fluid, cellular waste, and inflammatory proteins from tissues. After surgery, trauma to the tissues and lymph vessels leads to a significant increase in interstitial fluid (fluid between the tissues), contributing to swelling, tightness, and potential complications such as seroma or lymphedema (Mortimer & Rockson, 2014).

**Post-Surgical Swelling and Lymphatic Disruption**

Surgical trauma causes inflammation and fluid accumulation. Blood vessels become more permeable, allowing immune cells and plasma to flood the area. Meanwhile, lymphatic vessels, which are fragile and easily damaged during surgery, may be disrupted or overwhelmed. This mismatch between increased fluid production and reduced drainage capacity is the primary cause of post-surgical swelling. Gravity plays a role in swelling, too, pulling fluid downward causing tissue outside the surgical area to swell as well.

If left unmanaged, excessive swelling can lead to tissue hypoxia, delayed healing, increased risk of infection, and fibrosis. In aesthetic surgeries such as liposuction or tummy tucks, unmanaged lymphatic overload can alter surgical outcomes, creating contour irregularities or long-term firmness in the tissue.

**Clinical Importance of Lymphatic Support**

Lymphatic drainage techniques are essential for reducing fluid stagnation, promoting faster reabsorption of interstitial waste, and preventing complications. In one study, patients receiving manual lymphatic drainage (MLD) post-operatively demonstrated reduced limb circumference and faster return to function compared to controls (Leduc et al., 2009).

While manual lymphatic drainage (MLD) massage is a basic component of post-operative MLD, not all massage therapists are trained to provide safe post-operative lymphatic drainage. Post-operative care requires advanced understanding of the lymphatic system, tissue healing, scar tissue formation, and potential risks. Surgery alters the pathways of lymphatic movement, therefore, selecting a qualified provider with post-surgical experience and, ideally, wound care training, is critical.

**What is Manual Lymphatic Drainage (MLD)**

MLD is a gentle, rhythmic massage technique that encourages lymphatic fluid to move toward functioning lymph nodes. It uses light pressure and specific directional strokes to stimulate superficial lymph vessels just beneath the skin. Technique and direction of massage is critical and not like a relaxation massage.

**Important Consideration:** MLD should never be deep or painful. Deep pressure can damage fragile healing tissues and lymph vessels, particularly after procedures like liposuction. MLD does not use tools or creams, either. Movement of the skin is the most important factor in MLD massage, so use of tools or creams invalidates those critical techniques.

### Movement and Breathwork

Light movement and diaphragmatic breathing are essential companions to lymphatic therapy. The lymphatic system lacks its own pump and relies on compression and muscular contractions to move fluid. Walking and breathing deeply stimulate central lymph drainage and improve oxygen delivery to tissues.

Encouraging patients to walk every few hours and perform gentle breathwork, even while in bed, can dramatically improve lymph flow and reduce discomfort.

## Post-Operative Lymphatic Massage

Post-operative lymphatic massage differs significantly from traditional or deep tissue massage. It is a highly specialized, gentle technique aimed at supporting the lymphatic system without causing trauma to healing tissues.

For the first several weeks post-surgery, lymphatic drainage should always be performed using hands only, never with tools, machines, or cupping devices. The use of instruments during this delicate healing phase can be harmful and counterproductive. Likewise, no lotions or oils should be used during treatment, as they can interfere with the subtle skin-stretching motions required to effectively move lymphatic fluid.

The treatment is gentle, slow, and rhythmic. Patients often describe it as relaxing, but unlike traditional massage, there is no deep pressure, kneading, or muscle manipulation. Post-surgical MLD is also never performed with the client standing as gravity will defeat the treatment outcome. There are many stories of patients receiving postop MLD while standing, kneeling, on all fours, and other weird positions; this is a good indication the therapist is not properly trained in lymphatic flow and post-op recovery. For effective post-op MLD, the patient should be in a relaxed, horizontal position. The only exception is for recovery of procedures in the head and neck. Since the lymphatic outlets are "below" the face and neck, gravity is useful during this treatment.

It is important that patients are educated to avoid any provider who applies excessive pressure, require weird positioning, or causes pain during treatment.

**The Vodder Technique**

The Vodder Technique is one of the most respected and evidence-supported methods of manual lymphatic drainage. Developed in the 1930s by Dr. Emil Vodder and his wife Estrid, the method was originally designed to treat chronic sinusitis and other immune disorders by stimulating lymph flow. Today, it is widely practiced in clinical and post-surgical settings across the globe. MLD has been shown to effectively reduce edema and improve tissue recovery after orthopedic and cosmetic procedures (Hildebrandt et al., 2003).

The Vodder technique uses precise, gentle hand movements that stretch the skin in the direction of lymph flow, encouraging drainage from congested areas. Practitioners trained in the Vodder Method undergo extensive certification to ensure the safety and effectiveness of the treatment. Those practitioners who are working with post-operative patients should be trained further in post-operative MLD and wound care. Overall, post-op MLD is particularly effective in reducing post-operative swelling, preventing fibrosis, and improving patient comfort in the early stages of healing.

Patients seeking lymphatic massage should confirm that their provider is trained in the Vodder Technique or other certified MLD modality and that they understand the specific contraindications and adaptations required after surgery.

**How Surgery Changes the Lymphatic System**

Surgery, especially procedures involving the abdomen, breasts, or extremities, can significantly alter the body's lymphatic pathways. These changes occur when lymph vessels are severed, redirected, or obstructed due to incision lines, scar formation, or surgical removal of tissue. Because the lymphatic system operates in precise anatomical patterns, even minor disruptions can result in temporary or long-term congestion, swelling, or impaired drainage.

One example is abdominal surgery. In tummy tucks (abdominoplasty) and Cesarean sections, key superficial lymphatic pathways that normally drain toward the inguinal nodes may be interrupted. Research by Suami et al. (2017) using fluorescent lymphography imaging showed that post-abdominoplasty patients developed new collateral lymphatic pathways over time to compensate for disrupted flow, but this adaptation could take weeks or months. During this adaptation period, patients may experience prolonged swelling or tightness across the lower abdomen and flanks.

Cesarean sections also impact superficial and deep lymphatic vessels due to both the incision and uterine manipulation. Repetitive C-sections can increase the risk of scar tissue buildup and stagnant lymph flow, potentially contributing to sensations of pelvic heaviness, swelling, or discomfort during prolonged standing.

These structural changes underscore the importance of timely and skilled post-operative lymphatic drainage by well-trained therapists who understand the changes surgery forces on the body. Supporting lymph flow while the body rebuilds new pathways can reduce discomfort, minimize fibrosis, and improve surgical outcomes.

## Decongestive Therapy: Advanced Lymphatic Drainage Training

For patients requiring more advanced post-surgical or chronic swelling management, Complete Decongestive Therapy (CDT) may be recommended. CDT is the gold standard treatment for lymphedema and post-operative MLD. It includes advanced manual lymph drainage, compression bandaging, exercise, and skin care protocols. Therapists trained in decongestive therapy complete up to 170 hours of education and hands-on clinical training, far exceeding the baseline requirements for MLD certification.

This advanced training allows therapists to assess and treat more complex cases of lymphatic congestion, including patients recovering from cancer surgeries, lymph node removal, or individuals with pre-existing lymphatic compromise. It is also used preventatively for high-risk patients to avoid the onset of secondary lymphedema after surgery.

CDT-trained therapists are uniquely equipped to identify signs of fluid stagnation that may not respond to standard care. Their approach integrates medical-grade compression, scar tissue mobilization, and patient education for long-term management.

Post-operative patients experiencing persistent or recurrent swelling, fibrosis, or signs of lymphedema may benefit from working with a decongestive therapist in coordination with their surgeon. This partnership ensures optimal outcomes and helps reduce the risk of long-term complications.

## Recommended Frequency of Post-Surgical Lymphatic Massage

The frequency of post-operative lymphatic massage varies depending on the type of surgery, the amount of swelling, and individual healing response. While a general rule is to begin within 48 to 72 hours, many protocols support multiple sessions per week in the initial recovery phase. This section provides a guide for scheduling sessions based on surgery type.

| **Surgery Type** | **Week 1–2** | **Week 3–4** | **Week 5–6** | **Week 7-8** |
|---|---|---|---|---|
| Liposuction | 3–4 sessions/ week | 2–3 sessions/ week | 1–2 sessions/ week | As needed |
| Tummy Tuck (Abdominoplasty) | 2–4 sessions/ week | 2 sessions/ week | 1 session/ week | 1 session/ week |
| Breast Augmentation or Reduction | 2–3 sessions/ week | 1–2 sessions/ week | 1 session/ week | As needed |
| Facelift/Neck Lift | 2–3 gentle sessions/ week | 1–2 sessions/ week | 1–2 sessions/ week | 1 session/ week |
| Orthopedic Surgery | 2–3 sessions/ week | 2 sessions/ week | 1 session/ week | 1 session/ week |
| C-section or Gynecological | 2 sessions/ week | 1–2 sessions/ week | 1 session/ week | As needed |

These are guideline ranges and should be adjusted based on pain, swelling, bruising, and therapist/surgeon input. Patients should only work with trained post-operative massage professionals and avoid any painful or aggressive therapy as described earlier.

# Clinical Massage Therapy for Enhanced Recovery

Clinical massage therapy refers to advanced bodywork techniques applied by licensed therapists with medical knowledge and clinical experience. Unlike spa or relaxation massage, clinical therapy focuses on specific goals: reducing pain, improving mobility, preventing adhesions, and accelerating tissue healing. Clinical massage therapy is often used for joint and spine surgeries to facilitate ligament and tendon healing and is often incorporated into post-operative recovery during the later stages – after swelling has decreased and the joint or spine is becoming more stable.

**Addressing Tissue Adhesions and Fibrosis**

After surgery, especially with liposuction, abdominoplasty, or orthopedic procedures, the body forms fibrous adhesions as part of healing. These adhesions can restrict mobility, distort contours, and create chronic discomfort if they become excessive or disorganized.

Clinical massage therapists trained in post-op recovery use techniques such as myofascial release, cross-fiber friction, and scar tissue mobilization to break down early adhesions before they become problematic. Studies have shown that targeted manual therapy can reduce post-surgical stiffness and improve long-term range of motion (Schellenberger et al., 2007).

**Integrating Clinical Massage with Surgical Care**

An ideal post-surgical care team includes the surgeon, physical therapist, and clinical soft tissue therapist. Each plays a distinct role: the surgeon addresses structural repair, the physical therapist guides strength and mobility, and the clinical massage therapist works directly with soft tissues and the lymphatic system.

Evidence suggests that this multidisciplinary approach shortens recovery time and reduces post-operative complications such as stiffness, excessive scarring, and persistent swelling (Franklin et al., 2008).

**Note:** Therapists working with post-op patients should always communicate with the surgical team to ensure safety, especially when wound healing is ongoing or drains are in place.

**Cold Therapy and Elevation**

Cold packs can help reduce inflammation in the first 72 hours post-op, particularly for face and joint procedures. Elevating limbs above heart level also supports passive lymph drainage.

However, prolonged, or excessive cold use may slow lymph movement or numb healing nerves. Use intermittent cold applications with caution. Avoid ice only or frozen gel packs. The tissues will do just as well with a cold compress as it will with a frozen compress and you may save yourself from frostbite.

**Supporting the Nervous System and Emotional Recovery**

Beyond physical benefits, clinical manual soft tissue therapy can have a profound effect on the autonomic nervous system. Gentle massage has been shown to lower cortisol levels, reduce heart rate, and improve parasympathetic activity, the state associated with rest and repair (Field, 2014).

Many post-op patients experience anxiety, body image distress, or emotional lows in the weeks after surgery. Clinical massage offers not just physical touch, but therapeutic connection that can foster a sense of safety, confidence, and reconnection with the body.

## Conclusion

Lymphatic drainage and clinical manual soft tissue therapy are powerful allies in surgical recovery. By reducing swelling, preventing fibrosis, and supporting overall healing, these therapies enhance both the functional and aesthetic outcomes of surgery. While not all patients are informed of their value, those who include these modalities in their recovery often report faster healing, fewer complications, and improved satisfaction with their surgical results.

Patients are encouraged to seek out certified, experienced post-op therapists who understand the unique physiological needs of healing tissues. Surgeons and caregivers should also consider integrating lymphatic and clinical massage protocols into their standard aftercare plans for more holistic outcomes.

# Chapter 13

## Post-Op Scar Tissue Manipulation

Scar tissue is a natural part of the healing process, but it can present challenges during post-operative recovery. While the body's effort to mend tissue is essential, the resulting scar formation can sometimes inhibit movement, trap fluid, or disrupt normal lymphatic pathways. Integrating scar tissue manipulation into post-operative lymphatic drainage sessions can help reduce these complications and support better long-term outcomes.

Patients are typically unaware that post-operative scarring can create adhesions not just at the skin level, but deep within the fascia and connective tissues. These restrictions can contribute to stiffness, discomfort, uneven contours, and swelling which resists traditional methods of drainage. For this reason, trained manual therapists often incorporate scar tissue work as a critical part of holistic lymphatic recovery. By addressing adhesions early, once it is safe to do so, therapists can help restore mobility and prevent future complications.

This chapter explores how scars form, how they can impact healing and function, and how clinical practitioners integrate gentle manipulation into the broader scope of lymphatic recovery care.

## Why Scars Form and How They Develop

Scars form when the body repairs damaged skin and underlying tissues following injury or surgery. The healing process involves inflammation, proliferation, and remodeling. During the proliferative phase, fibroblasts produce large amounts of collagen, a structural protein, to close and strengthen the wound. Unlike the basket-weave pattern of normal skin, scar tissue collagen is laid down in a more linear, dense, and less elastic formation.

This new tissue is essential for wound integrity, but it is less flexible and lacks the functionality of original skin. Scar tissue is typically void of sweat glands, hair follicles, and the full nerve supply found in healthy skin. Over time, the body enters a remodeling phase in which collagen alignment and tensile strength are gradually refined, sometimes for up to two years. However, depending on individual healing capacity, skin tone, surgical site, and aftercare, some scars may become problematic.

In certain individuals, scar formation becomes exaggerated or poorly organized. When the body overproduces collagen or heals too quickly, it may result in raised or dense scars which limit tissue mobility. In surgeries involving multiple layers, such as tummy tucks or breast reductions, adhesions can form between layers of fascia, skin, and muscle, restricting range of motion and impeding lymphatic flow. Proactive care during healing can mitigate these outcomes.

Not every clinical soft tissue therapist is comfortable working with scar tissue and many times scar tissue is ignored until it is too late. Post-surgical care is as much about technique as it is about timing. Treat too early and wounds may open, scars may widen. Treat too late and wounds will be stiff, treatments will be more painful. Well qualified therapists will recognize when it is appropriate to treat the scar and with the proper technique.  Don't be afraid to ask your therapist detailed questions. With the information presented in this chapter, you may know more than they do!

## Common Scar Types and Characteristics

Understanding scar types helps guide appropriate treatment. Below is a table outlining common types of scars seen in post-operative patients.

| Scar Type | Appearance | Clinical Notes |
|---|---|---|
| Normal (Mature) | Flat, pale or flesh-colored, blends with skin tone | Forms over 12–18 months, non-problematic |
| Hypertrophic | Raised, firm, red or pink, within surgical borders | May regress over time; often itchy or tight |
| Keloid | Raised, extends beyond incision borders, dark or discolored | More common in darker skin types; prone to recurrence |
| Atrophic | Sunken or pitted, often from trauma or infections | May appear as indented lines or folds |
| Adhesive | Bound to deeper layers, restricts movement, or causes discomfort | Common post-cosmetic surgery; may interfere with lymphatic drainage |

Hypertrophic scars and adhesions are among the most common concerns after surgery and are often responsive to therapeutic intervention. Keloids require special consideration and are typically managed with medical oversight, but gentle massage may help reduce discomfort and support skin mobility.

Atrophic scars, while less common in surgery, may occur following wound infections or in individuals with compromised collagen production. C-section scars often appear atrophic but are following the natural folds of skin in the lower abdomen. Atrophic scars are best treated with a combination of manual techniques, topical therapies, and, if necessary, dermatologic intervention.

## Integrating Scar Manipulation into Lymphatic Massage

Scar tissue manipulation during post-op lymphatic massage must be approached with caution and skill. These techniques are never applied in the first few days or when a wound is open, weeping, or not fully sealed. Typically, direct scar work begins around 3–6 weeks post-op, depending on incision healing and the complexity of surgery. Scar mobility work can begin as soon as 3-days post-op. The difference being scar mobility work is very gentle movement of the tissue to avoid adhesion to underlying tissues and direct scar work is more aggressive on the scar itself. If the therapist is not trained in scar work, they should avoid the scar during any treatments.

In the early stages of integration, therapists begin by gently mobilizing the tissues surrounding the scar. This includes directional strokes along the edges of the incision, light skin movement, and rhythmic motions designed to enhance lymph movement without directly stressing the scar. These movements encourage healthy circulation and reduce the risk of fluid stagnation around healing tissue.

As healing progresses and the scar becomes more stable, direct manipulation can be safely introduced. This includes skin rolling, longitudinal friction (in the same direction as the scar), gentle pinching and lifting, and light compression. The goal is not to "break" scar tissue but to soften it gradually and support the reorganization of collagen fibers. These techniques are especially useful in preventing the development of hard, ropey, or painful adhesions which can interfere with normal lymphatic drainage.

When done consistently, this combined approach, lymphatic drainage followed by targeted scar tissue work, can produce superior outcomes in terms of comfort, mobility, and aesthetics. Therapists often note scar manipulation improves drainage efficiency by reducing mechanical barriers in the tissue.

## Surgery-Specific Scar Formation and Sensations

Different surgical procedures result in varying types of incisions, tissue disruption, and scar characteristics. Understanding how scars form and feel depending on the surgery type can guide treatment and patient expectations.

**Liposuction**

Liposuction scars are typically small (5–10 mm) but can become surrounded by fibrous nodules beneath the surface, often referred to as fibrosis. While the incision itself may heal quickly, the underlying scar tissue from cannula movement and fat extraction can lead to hardened areas that feel like lumps or bands under the skin. According to Rohrich et al. (2006), post-liposuction fibrosis is a frequent cause of patient dissatisfaction and is best addressed with early soft tissue work and myofascial mobilization.

**Abdominoplasty (Tummy Tuck)**

Abdominoplasty results in a long, horizontal scar along the lower abdomen and sometimes a circular scar around the navel and sometimes a deeper scar for diastasis recti repair. Because this area involves extensive undermining of the skin and fascia, adhesions are common and can limit core mobility. Patients often report tightness or pulling when standing or stretching. Research by Lee and Mun (2013) indicates that targeted scar massage and mobilization during the first six months post-op improve range of motion and aesthetic results significantly.

**Knee Replacement or Repair**

Knee surgery scars may develop adhesions that restrict joint flexion and extension. The scar runs vertically over the patella and can become bound to the underlying fascia and joint capsule. Patients frequently experience stiffness, heat, and scar pain with movement. A study by Kim et al. (2018) found that scar massage as part of physical therapy accelerated range-of-motion gains and reduced subjective pain scores within 12 weeks post-op. Additional scaring is frequently noticed under the skin in the areas of surgery – in the ligaments and tendons. Scar tissue manipulation in these areas can often improve mobility and range of motion sooner.

**Deep Plane Face/Neck Lift**

This complex facial procedure involves incisions around the ears, hairline, and under the chin. These scars often heal discreetly but may cause stiffness in the platysma muscle or pull at facial expressions if adhesions form. Patients report sensations of numbness, skin tethering, or localized hardness near suture lines. Delicate scar work, starting 3–6 weeks post-op, can restore natural tissue glide and reduce visible irregularities. Chia et al. (2015) highlight that skilled scar treatment improves facial contour and reduces long-term textural changes. Since skin on the face and neck is very thin, it is extremely important that only qualified and well-trained manual soft tissue therapists be allowed to work in this area.

**Brazilian Butt Lift (BBL)**

BBL surgery involves liposuction of fat from areas such as the abdomen, flanks, or thighs, followed by fat transfer to the buttocks. Scars from liposuction are typically small and scattered, while fat injection sites may leave minimal surface evidence. However, internal trauma and cannula movement can lead to fibrosis and uneven texture. According to Cárdenas-Camarena et al. (2015), post-liposuction fibrosis in BBL patients can be particularly challenging due to tissue density in the gluteal region. While massage of fat augmentation areas is typically avoided, manual therapy around any fibrotic areas can help soften these areas and improve lymphatic movement, especially during the first three months post-op. As with ant fat augmentation, additional scar tissue formation can occur months or even a year after the injection. These scars are often nodular (small or large) and can be tender or painful as they adhere to the underlying tissue. Scar treatment can be effective but often uncomfortable as the fascial adhesions are released.

**Mastectomy (Breast Removal Surgery)**

Mastectomy, the surgical removal of one or both breasts, is often performed as part of breast cancer treatment. This procedure can lead to large, firm scars across the chest wall, especially when combined with lymph node removal or radiation therapy. Scars from mastectomy may feel tight, numb, or hypersensitive, and the emotional weight of such a procedure can also impact a patient's relationship with their body. When a patient allows an oncology-trained manual soft tissue therapist to work on the scars and chest tissue, this touch can help restore confidence in their body. Ask the therapist to teach you some of the maintenance techniques you can do at home!

In cases where tissue expanders or immediate reconstruction are not performed, mastectomy scars may also become tethered to the underlying pectoralis muscle and ribcage. Scar mobilization in these cases must be gentle and focused on restoring mobility, reducing restriction during shoulder or torso movement, and helping the patient reconnect with their healing body. Cheville et al. (2001) emphasizes the importance of multidisciplinary rehabilitation, including scar work and lymphatic support, for post-mastectomy patients.

**Breast Reconstruction After Cancer Treatment**

Breast reconstruction after mastectomy or lumpectomy often involves extensive scar formation, flap procedures, or implant-based reconstruction. These patients may also have scars from lymph node dissection, which can interfere with lymphatic flow. According to Cheville et al. (2001), scar adhesion in axillary or chest wall regions can contribute to pain, swelling, and limited shoulder mobility. Gentle scar tissue manipulation can significantly improve range of motion, reduce discomfort, and support emotional healing in this population.

**Breast Lift**

Breast lifts typically result in a scar under each breast, another scar vertical from under the breast to the areola, and a third scar around the areola – collectively called an "anchor scar." Breast lifts are a reduction in breast size and in some cases, alignment. Most often the areola and nipple tissue along with the "stem" is relocated as tissue underneath the breast is removed. Incisions under the breast are the most delicate and should be protected. The scars from a breast lift, with or without implants, will typically cause adhesion in axillary or chest wall regions and can contribute to pain, swelling, and limited shoulder mobility. Gentle scar tissue manipulation can significantly improve range of motion, reduce discomfort, and support emotional healing. Additionally, certain movements of the breast implant are necessary to avoid cording or capsulation as the tissue heals. Clinical manual soft tissue therapy by a qualified, well-trained therapists is essential during the healing process.

**Thigh Lift**

Thigh lifts typically result in long incisions along the inner thigh or groin area. These scars are prone to friction, moisture, and tension, which can increase the likelihood of hypertrophic scarring and delayed healing. Patients often report tightness when walking or sitting. A study by Fruhstorfer et al. (2013) supports early intervention with scar massage to reduce tethering and improve comfort. Therapists should approach these areas with sensitivity due to the potential for tenderness and nerve involvement.

## Benefits and Outcomes

When done properly, scar manipulation can:

- Improve lymphatic drainage and reduce local swelling
- Increase range of motion in affected areas
- Minimize sensations of tightness, itching, or burning
- Improve cosmetic appearance and surgical contour
- Support emotional healing and reintegration

Clinical studies show that scar massage, especially when introduced within the first three months post-op, improves scar pliability, vascularization, and patient satisfaction (Cho et al., 2014). Patients often report decreased tenderness and improved sensation in areas previously affected by scarring. In procedures involving large or circumferential scars, like abdominoplasty, consistent therapy may also reduce the risk of fibrosis and fluid pockets.

Beyond physical benefits, scar manipulation can support emotional and psychological healing. Many patients describe a sense of disconnection from areas that have undergone surgery. Scar massage, delivered with care and education, allows individuals to reclaim comfort, awareness, and autonomy in their own bodies. This therapeutic relationship fosters trust and confidence during what can otherwise be a vulnerable stage of recovery.

## Special Considerations and Contraindications

While scar work is widely beneficial, it must be adapted to the patient's surgical history and healing timeline. Contraindications include open wounds, active infections, skin grafts not yet integrated, and untreated keloids. Therapists must also be cautious with patients who have compromised skin integrity, bleeding disorders, or uncontrolled diabetes.

In patients with known lymphedema, scar tissue manipulation should only be performed by therapists trained in Complete Decongestive Therapy (CDT) or equivalent programs. These specialists understand how to safely work around fragile lymphatic territories and incorporate compression protocols when needed.

Clear communication with the surgical team is also essential. Surgeons can advise when scars are mature enough for manual intervention and provide insight into any complications that may influence treatment decisions.

# Conclusion

Scar tissue is a natural part of healing, but it does not have to interfere with recovery. With informed, skilled scar tissue manipulation, integrated into manual lymphatic drainage therapy, patients can enjoy smoother healing, better cosmetic outcomes, and fewer long-term restrictions. When combined with education, breathwork, and therapeutic rapport, scar therapy becomes more than a technique, it becomes an empowering part of the recovery journey.

As this field continues to grow, more patients and providers recognize the value of early, safe scar work to restore function and foster resilience. Therapists trained in post-operative care and scar dynamics are well positioned to offer this integrative service with confidence and compassion.

# Chapter 14

## Mental Health & Emotional Recovery

Surgical recovery involves more than just physical healing. Emotional and psychological shifts are common following cosmetic and reconstructive procedures. Patients may feel joy and relief, but also experience uncertainty, sadness, and frustration. Understanding the emotional arc of recovery and having tools for support can make a significant difference in healing outcomes and long-term satisfaction.

This chapter explores common post-operative emotional challenges, changes in body image, and evidence-based strategies for stress management and emotional resilience. Addressing mental health is not only about mitigating challenges but also about empowering patients to embrace their new appearance, restore confidence, and feel supported throughout their transformation.

### Coping with Post-Operative Blues

It is not uncommon for patients to experience a dip in mood in the days and weeks following surgery. Known as the "post-op blues," this temporary emotional slump may include feelings of sadness, regret, irritability, or anxiety. These emotions are often compounded by pain, physical limitations, and the inability to perform daily tasks independently. The sudden disruption of routine, along with time spent isolated during rest, can increase feelings of vulnerability.

According to a study by Sarwer et al. (2005), while most patients are satisfied with cosmetic outcomes, the early recovery period can trigger doubts and emotional discomfort, especially when swelling, bruising, and pain distort expectations. It is crucial to normalize these feelings and remind patients that emotional lows are a normal part of healing.

Sleep disruption, medication side effects, hormonal changes, and temporary loss of independence can also influence mood. Supportive conversations with care providers, family, or therapists can help patients process their emotions and navigate recovery more comfortably. In some cases, patients may benefit from a temporary adjustment of mood-regulating medication or scheduled check-ins with a mental health professional.

Social support has helped to buffer the effects of surgical stress. One study found that patients who had access to consistent emotional support reported less pain, better coping, and faster healing (Kiecolt-Glaser et al., 2005). Engaging in regular dialogue with loved ones or simply having a consistent support person to assist with daily tasks, can greatly improve emotional stability.

Recognizing that these symptoms are typically short-lived, and often resolve as the body heals. However, persistent sadness, lack of interest in daily activities, or thoughts of hopelessness should always be taken seriously and brought to the attention of a qualified mental health professional.

## Body Image and Adjusting to Changes

Cosmetic and reconstructive surgeries often bring dramatic physical changes. While many patients anticipate these outcomes with excitement, the reality of seeing one's altered body for the first time can be jarring. Swelling, bruising, and asymmetry are common early on and may interfere with body image and confidence. Temporary changes in posture, body fluid shifts, or compression garments may further distort self-perception.

A study by von Soest et al. (2006) found that while most cosmetic surgery patients reported improved body image in the long term, many also experienced a temporary decline in satisfaction immediately post-op. Emotional adjustment takes time, and it is important for patients to understand that healing is a process, not just of the body, but of self-perception.

Some individuals may experience body dysmorphia or struggle with feeling disconnected from their new appearance. In such cases, professional counseling or body image therapy can help patients integrate the changes and foster self-acceptance. Open communication with a trusted provider can also ease concerns, especially if the patient feels anxious about results during the early healing stages.

Visual desensitization, where patients are slowly reintroduced to viewing their body, can be a useful technique. Gradual exposure to mirrors, journaling, photography, and positive affirmations can also aid emotional adaptation. Providers should encourage patients to approach body image with curiosity and kindness rather than criticism. Celebrating small signs of healing and documenting progress over time may also shift focus from imperfections to achievements.

Developing a healthy relationship with one's appearance after surgery involves learning to accept natural asymmetries, shifting expectations, and reimagining beauty standards. Emotional integration of physical change can take weeks or even months, and patients should not feel pressured to "love" their new body immediately. Instead, focus on curiosity, compassion, and patience.

## Phases of Emotional Trauma Recovery

Emotional healing after surgery often mirrors the psychological process seen in trauma recovery. While the surgical event may be planned and elective, the physical trauma, anesthesia, and post-operative pain can trigger a deep emotional response that patients are not always prepared for. Understanding the stages of trauma recovery can help normalize the emotional journey.

**1. Denial**

Initially, patients may experience a disconnect from the surgical event. They might minimize discomfort, avoid acknowledging difficult emotions, or feel emotionally numb. This is a protective response to overwhelming change and uncertainty.

**2. Bargaining**

As physical symptoms emerge, patients may try to mentally negotiate with themselves or their healing process. Thoughts like, "If I rest for one more day, I'll look perfect by the weekend," are common. This phase reflects an attempt to regain control over a body that feels unfamiliar.

**3. Depression**

As the reality of discomfort, appearance changes, and limitations setting in, some patients may experience sadness, withdrawal, or hopelessness. They may question their decision to have had surgery. This stage often peaks around the 1–2 week mark when physical healing feels slowest.

**4. Anger**

Frustration with the pace of healing, dependency on others, or unmet expectations can trigger anger. Patients might feel resentful toward their care team, loved ones, or themselves. Validating these feelings and offering tools for expression is important.

**5. Acceptance**

Gradually, most patients begin to see progress. Swelling subsides, strength returns, and they start to feel more like themselves. Acceptance does not always mean full contentment, but it does signal a willingness to adapt, heal, and move forward with a new sense of identity.

These stages are fluid and may overlap or repeat. Not all patients experience every stage, and emotional support throughout this process is critical. Providers should help patients name their feelings, offer reassurance, and direct them to therapeutic resources when needed.

## What to Expect in the Mirror: Week-by-Week Appearance Changes

Seeing oneself after surgery can be emotionally intense. The mirror often reflects temporary side effects like swelling, bruising, incisions, or asymmetry that may not match a patient's expectations. Preparing for these stages can help patients approach the healing process with compassion and patience.

### Week 1

During the first week, swelling and bruising are at their peak. The face, abdomen, limbs, or surgical area may appear significantly distorted. Patients may see deep discoloration (purples, blues, and yellows), puffiness, and prominent surgical tape or drains. According to Klinger et al. (2018), early-phase inflammation and trauma to the tissues result in altered body perception and emotional vulnerability. It is important for patients to limit mirror exposure if it triggers distress.

### Week 2

By the second week, bruising begins to fade, changing to green or yellow tones. Swelling may still be prominent, but some definition returns. Sutures may be removed, and bandages reduced. Patients may feel slightly more hopeful as early signs of healing become visible, though asymmetries or uneven swelling can remain. Research from Sarwer and Crerand (2004) emphasizes that visible healing milestones often correlate with improved mood and satisfaction.

### Week 3–4

The body continues to reabsorb fluids, and overall appearance starts to settle. At this stage, patients begin to recognize early contours of their surgical outcomes. However, residual swelling, hardness, or firmness in tissues is still normal. Skin texture may appear tight or shiny, and numbness around incisions can persist. Many patients experience a "rollercoaster" of emotions during this period as they compare expectations to current appearance.

### Week 5–8

Most major bruising is gone, and swelling decreases significantly. Scars may look pink or raised but begin softening. This is when patients often feel a renewed connection to their bodies and can better appreciate the results. According to Reavey et al. (2011), positive shifts in body image typically increase around the two-month mark as physical changes stabilize.

### Beyond Week 8

Appearance continues to improve gradually over several months. Scar fading, continued tissue remodeling, and minor symmetry adjustments occur. By 3–6 months, most patients see a stable version of their surgical outcome, though some residual swelling may persist. Emotional reactions vary, some feel empowered and satisfied, while others may still struggle with unexpected outcomes. Continued support and monitoring remain important.

Understanding this timeline helps set realistic expectations. Patients are encouraged to document progress through photos and track emotional shifts as part of the recovery journey.

## Stress-Reducing Techniques for Recovery

Recovery can be physically and emotionally taxing. Integrating stress-reducing practices into daily routines helps calm the nervous system, improve sleep, and support faster healing. Many of these techniques are free, accessible, and can be done from the comfort of the recovery space.

**1. Breathwork and Meditation:**

Deep, diaphragmatic breathing has been shown to reduce cortisol levels and shift the body into a parasympathetic state, which promotes tissue repair and emotional calm (Brown & Gerbarg, 2005). Guided meditations or body scans can also help patients reconnect with their bodies and reduce anxiety. Apps such as Calm, Insight Timer, or Headspace provide easily accessible resources for beginners.

**2. Gentle Movement:**

When appropriate, light stretching, short walks, or restorative yoga poses can reduce muscle tension, improve circulation, and enhance mood through endorphin release. Movement also contributes to lymphatic flow, reducing post-op swelling. Always consult a medical provider before resuming physical activity, but even small steps, like changing positions in bed regularly, can benefit mental clarity.

**3. Creative Expression:**

Art, music, journaling, or other creative outlets offer a constructive way to process feelings during recovery. Expressive therapies have been linked to improved coping and reduced depressive symptoms (Stuckey & Nobel, 2010). Patients may benefit from drawing their healing journey, writing reflective notes, or engaging in crafts to pass time and reduce ruminative thoughts.

**4. Therapy and Support Groups:**

Speaking with a licensed counselor or joining a support group of others who have undergone similar procedures can reduce feelings of isolation and provide validation during the healing journey. Online forums, virtual support meetings, or in-person gatherings can be great tools for building community. Be careful of social media group chatter – healing is different for everyone.

**5. Sleep Hygiene and Routine:**

Creating a calming evening routine can enhance sleep quality, a critical factor in both physical and emotional recovery. Avoid screens before bed, dim the lights, and use calming rituals such as reading, lavender essential oil, or herbal teas. Consistent sleep routines stabilize mood and support healing.

**6. Nutrition and Hydration:**

Though discussed in earlier chapters, it's worth emphasizing that balanced nutrition plays a key role in mental health. Deficiencies in nutrients like vitamin D, B12, and magnesium are associated with mood disturbances. Staying hydrated and nourished can improve energy levels and overall outlook.

Patients who engage in mindfulness or self-care practices during recovery often report improved outcomes and satisfaction. Encouraging even small daily habits, like drinking tea mindfully, sitting in sunlight, or listening to calming music, can make a noticeable difference.

# Chapter 15

## Long-Term Maintenance and Beauty Tips

Long-term recovery and satisfaction after cosmetic surgery rely on consistent care, realistic expectations, and proactive strategies. While the initial weeks are critical for healing, the months and years following surgery are equally important for preserving results, nurturing skin health, and knowing when professional evaluation might be needed.

Many patients mistakenly believe that surgery produces permanent results without upkeep, but the truth is that aging, lifestyle habits, sun exposure, and overall health all play significant roles in how surgical outcomes evolve. In fact, long-term satisfaction depends on a patient's willingness to adopt sustainable beauty and wellness habits. This chapter explores how to maintain surgical outcomes, implement post-procedure skincare routines, and assess when revision surgery might be considered.

### Maintaining Surgical Results

The longevity of cosmetic surgery results depends on a combination of surgical technique, genetics, lifestyle, and patient adherence to aftercare. Procedures like liposuction, facelifts, tummy tucks, and breast augmentation yield excellent results, but those results can shift over time due to factors such as aging, hormonal changes, gravity, and fluctuations in weight.

Maintaining a stable weight is one of the most important factors for preserving surgical outcomes. For example, weight gain after liposuction can cause fat to return in untreated areas or even develop unevenly, leading to contour irregularities.

Regular exercise, a healthy diet, and body composition monitoring are essential. According to Rohrich et al. (2008), long-term patient satisfaction after body contouring procedures was significantly higher in patients who adopted lifestyle changes to support their results.

Cardiovascular and strength-training exercise contribute not only to overall health but also to improved skin tone and metabolism, which help maintain surgical contours. Resistance training can be particularly effective in sustaining the lifted appearance achieved through body contouring. Similarly, posture-focused exercises like yoga or Pilates may enhance the appearance of surgical results in the abdomen and upper body.

Sun protection also plays a key role in maintaining outcomes, especially for procedures involving the face. UV exposure accelerates skin aging, increases pigmentation irregularities, and can even affect the integrity of surgical scars. Patients should use a broad-spectrum SPF 30 or higher daily, reapply sunscreen throughout the day, and wear hats or protective clothing during prolonged outdoor activities.

Additionally, scar care should continue well after wounds have closed. The use of silicone sheeting, scar massage, and topical antioxidants can improve the appearance of surgical scars and prevent thickening or hyperpigmentation. Scheduling annual follow-ups with a surgeon can also help monitor healing and identify any early signs of changes in surgical results.

Compression garments, scar care regimens, lymphatic drainage, and touch-up procedures such as Botox, dermal fillers, or skin resurfacing treatments may help enhance or maintain results. While not every patient requires these adjuncts, many benefit from a personalized plan that evolves with their lifestyle and goals.

## Skincare Routines After Cosmetic Procedures

Proper skincare following cosmetic surgery is vital for healing and long-term beauty. The skin experiences trauma during surgery, and tailored skincare supports recovery while minimizing complications like infection, hyperpigmentation, and scarring.

In the immediate post-op period, gentle cleansing with non-fragranced, non-foaming cleansers helps keep incisions clean without stripping natural oils. Moisturizers containing ceramides or hyaluronic acid support barrier repair and reduce transepidermal water loss. These ingredients also help soothe inflammation and provide hydration without causing irritation. Topicals with vitamin C or niacinamide may be introduced once the skin is fully closed to aid in collagen formation and brightening, while also offering antioxidant protection.

As healing progresses, incorporating ingredients like peptides, panthenol, and licorice extract can support skin elasticity and reduce post-inflammatory discoloration. Retinoids and exfoliants should be avoided until cleared by a provider, as they can irritate sensitive or healing skin. Once healed, retinoid use can stimulate collagen remodeling and reduce scar thickness. A study by Kang et al. (2005) showed that consistent use of topical retinoids significantly improved skin texture and minimized visible signs of aging.

Facial cosmetic procedures like facelifts, rhinoplasty, or blepharoplasty benefit from targeted regimens that focus on hydration, barrier repair, and UV protection. For example, patients might use a hydrating mask two to three times per week or apply growth factor serums that promote cellular regeneration. According to Mustoe et al. (2002), these types of topical treatments can significantly reduce the severity and duration of scarring.

For body surgeries, silicone sheets, scar gels, and daily scar massage can reduce hypertrophic scarring and promote smoother skin texture. Applying products twice daily for 2–3 months post-surgery often yields optimal results. Professional-grade treatments, including microneedling, fractional lasers, or enzyme peels, may be appropriate after the six month mark for patients seeking to refine the skin's surface and reduce scar visibility.

Routine professional skincare, such as medical facials or laser treatments, may also help maintain results and keep the skin vibrant over time. Annual skin evaluations by a dermatologist or licensed esthetician can ensure patients are using the best products for their evolving skin needs.

## Understanding Ingredients in Post-Surgical Topicals

Incorporating the right topical product is essential for supporting skin recovery after cosmetic surgery. These products work not only to protect the skin but also to enhance moisture retention, reduce inflammation, fade discoloration, and support collagen production. Below is a breakdown of commonly recommended active ingredients and their roles in the post-operative skincare regimen.

**Hyaluronic Acid**
Hyaluronic acid (HA) is a powerful humectant that draws water into the skin, helping to keep it plump, hydrated, and supple. Post-operatively, it helps improve barrier function and accelerates epithelial repair, especially when the skin is dry or irritated. HA-based serums or moisturizers are typically safe for all skin types and can be used early in recovery to improve comfort and reduce tightness (Rawlings & Harding, 2004).

**Peptides**
Peptides are small chains of amino acids that serve as messengers to the skin, promoting collagen synthesis and tissue repair. In post-surgical care, they can help reduce inflammation, improve elasticity, and assist in wound remodeling. Certain peptides, such as Matrixyl (palmitoyl pentapeptide), have been shown to reduce the depth of wrinkles and improve skin firmness over time (Lodén & Maibach, 2009).

**Retinol (Vitamin A Derivative)**

Retinol is a gold standard ingredient for increasing cell turnover and boosting collagen production. However, it should only be introduced after 3-4 months post-op, when incisions are fully healed, as it can be irritating. When appropriate, retinol helps soften scars, blend skin tone, and improve surface texture. Studies confirm regular retinoid use improves overall skin quality and reduces photoaging (Kang et al., 2005).

**Camphor and Menthol**

These ingredients are often found in post-surgical gels or creams designed to soothe itching, bruising, or discomfort. Camphor has mild anesthetic and antimicrobial properties, while menthol provides a cooling sensation that can alleviate post-op itchiness. However, these ingredients should not be used on open wounds and are best suited for mature scars or areas with minor swelling (Andersen, 2001).

**Dimethicone (Silicone-Based)**

Dimethicone is a form of silicone frequently used in scar treatments and barrier creams. It helps form a breathable seal over the skin, maintaining moisture and reducing transepidermal water loss. It also minimizes friction and helps scars appear smoother over time. Silicone-based topicals, such as gels or sheets, are a mainstay of scar prevention and have been supported by robust clinical evidence (Mustoe et al., 2002).

**Niacinamide**

Niacinamide, also known as vitamin B3, is a versatile active ingredient known for its calming, brightening, and anti-inflammatory properties. After surgery, niacinamide can help reduce redness, fade hyperpigmentation, and support the skin barrier by increasing ceramide production. It is well-tolerated by most skin types and can be used in both early and long-term post-operative skincare. Research shows niacinamide's efficacy in reducing fine lines, skin discoloration, and improving overall skin elasticity (Draelos, 2013).

**Panthenol**

Panthenol (provitamin B5) is hydrating and soothing with humectant properties, meaning it helps draw moisture into the skin. It enhances wound healing by improving epidermal barrier function and reducing transepidermal water loss. Post-surgical skin, which may be sensitive and dry, can benefit from panthenol-containing products. A study by Ebner et al. (2002) found that topical panthenol significantly improved skin hydration and softness during recovery.

**Retinoids**

Retinoids are a class of compounds derived from vitamin A, including retinol, tretinoin, and retinaldehyde. While retinol has already been discussed, it is worth noting that prescription-strength retinoids like tretinoin are more potent and may offer enhanced benefits in collagen remodeling and scar reduction, once healing is complete. These agents accelerate cell turnover and are supported by decades of dermatological research for anti-aging and scar care. Patients should be advised to introduce retinoids slowly and with proper sun protection.

**Sunscreen (Broad-Spectrum SPF)**

Daily sun protection is critical after surgery. UVA and UVB rays can darken scars, delay healing, and accelerate skin aging. Broad-spectrum sunscreens protect the skin while it is vulnerable and help prevent hyperpigmentation around surgical sites. Physical sunscreens with zinc oxide or titanium dioxide are often better tolerated post-surgery. The American Academy of Dermatology recommends SPF 30 or higher for patients recovering from any skin trauma (AAD, 2020).

Choosing high-quality formulations tailored to individual skin type and surgical procedure ensures the safest and most effective healing. Patients should consult with their provider to determine when each ingredient can be introduced based on their specific recovery stage.

## When to Consider Revision Surgery

Revision surgery refers to additional procedures performed to correct or improve the results of an initial surgery. It can be part of the normal aesthetic journey or arise due to complications, dissatisfaction, or natural changes over time.

Patients should wait until full healing is complete, typically 6–12 months, before evaluating the outcome. Swelling, scar maturation, and tissue settling all influence the final look. According to Tanna and Patel (2017), premature revision decisions often result from unrealistic early expectations or lack of awareness about healing timelines.

Reasons for revision may include asymmetry, under- or over-correction, scar visibility, poor healing, capsular contracture (in the case of implants), or changes related to aging. Some patients also seek revision to refine or enhance their original results, even if the first surgery healed as expected. These goals may include subtle contour adjustments, scar revisions, or the addition of new procedures to complement existing outcomes.

When considering revision, patients should work with an experienced and board-certified surgeon who specializes in the relevant procedure. A detailed consultation should include an honest discussion of goals, risks, healing history, and options. A new surgical plan should consider prior scar tissue, healing patterns, and emotional readiness.

In some cases, non-surgical treatments like laser resurfacing, radiofrequency tightening, or filler injections may provide satisfactory results without the need for additional surgery. Providers should help patients weigh the pros and cons of surgical vs. non-surgical revision options.

It is important for patients to understand that second surgeries often carry higher risks due to scar tissue, disrupted anatomy, or altered blood supply. The psychological component of revision should also be addressed, patients may feel disappointed or anxious, and compassionate communication is key. In cases where revision is not advisable, patients should be supported in embracing their current results and guided toward realistic, body-positive outcomes.

# Chapter 16

## Compression Garments and Adjuncts

Post-operative recovery involves more than surgical healing, supportive care tools like compression garments and adjuncts play a crucial role in comfort, swelling reduction, tissue shaping, and overall outcomes. These garments and devices are not one-size-fits-all and are typically prescribed or recommended based on the type of procedure, healing stage, and patient needs.

Understanding the timing, types, and purpose of each garment or adjunct can make a major difference in healing results and patient comfort. This chapter outlines why compression garments are effective, introduces key adjunct tools used after specific surgeries, and includes a table outlining the recommended use timeline for popular garments. It also explains best practices for wearing and maintaining these garments throughout the healing journey.

### Why Compression Garments Work

Compression garments apply consistent, gentle pressure to healing tissues. This external pressure helps minimize swelling (edema), reduces bruising, supports tissue adhesion, and enhances lymphatic drainage. Compression also helps reduce the risk of fluid collection, such as seromas, and improves the overall contour as tissues settle.

Compression and binding has been used for thousands of years to promote changes to the body with and without surgery. Many know of foot binding in China and the use of corsets during the Victorian era. In these instances, compression may have been done with or without a surgical procedure. Today, compression is a staple in supporting or fixating areas of the body for healing – usually as a result of trauma or surgery.

The physiological mechanism of compression is multifaceted. It encourages microcirculation, promotes the reabsorption of extracellular fluids, and provides external support to weakened or inflamed tissue structures. These effects collectively help reduce inflammation and improve tissue remodeling.

According to Matarasso and Wallach (2005), compression improves comfort, reduces post-op complications, and supports better scar maturation. These garments stabilize the surgical site, preventing undue stress from movement or tension and helping patients resume daily activity with more ease. In procedures involving large areas such as the abdomen, thighs, or buttocks, compression can dramatically reduce recovery time by supporting structural realignment.

Properly fitted compression garments also reduce pain and the sensation of "heaviness" that some patients feel after procedures like liposuction, abdominoplasty, or Brazilian butt lifts. A well-designed garment helps patients feel more secure when moving, and it reduces the risk of postural changes which can occur from guarding sore areas. Continuous use during the first few weeks after surgery is widely supported in the literature for optimal outcomes. Since the body does not store air, compression can also limit dead space, which reduces fluid accumulation.

## What is a Faja?

Compression garments come in various styles – waistbands, vest style, jacket-style, bodysuit style (as shorts, capri, or long legs) and bike shorts style. In many places, these are often referred to simply as "Fajas" (pronounced: ˈfä(ˌ)hä), but the dictionary defines a Faja as a waistband or girdle. Just to be a bit more confusing, waistbands are often referred to as waist-trainers or binders, too. What is needed for compression in any one area is often dictated by the type of procedure and the area of the body.

When discussing compression garments, remember there are three stages of compression for post-op care.

- **Stage 1:** Garments for Stage 1 are typically looser, easier to apply, and used within the first few days post-op to accommodate swelling. Stage 1 garments are often single layer, slip on or have a zipper, and they are somewhat stretchy.

- **Stage 2:** About 1-2 weeks post-op, a Stage 2 garment should be worn. Stage 2 garments are more form-fitting, not as stretchy, typically come with 1-3 columns of clips for closure, and can be double-walled for strength and compression. Stage 2 garments are used once swelling begins to subside and are typically worn through week eight or longer.

- **Stage 3:** Some patients transition to Stage 3 garments which offer lighter compression but are still helpful for long-term contour support. These garments are sometimes referred to as shapewear.

## Adjuncts for Specific Areas

In addition to compression garments, adjuncts like abdominal boards, back boards, genital pads, and foam inserts are often recommended depending on the surgery and the swelling. These tools add targeted pressure, fill anatomical voids, and prevent creases or fluid pockets during healing. When used correctly, they improve symmetry and promote smooth contours.

- **Abdominal boards** are rigid inserts placed under fajas or binders to prevent fluid build-up and contour the abdominal wall. They provide even pressure and help shape the waist post-liposuction or tummy tuck. Abdominal boards are usually introduced around day 4–7 and worn until week 4–6 depending on patient tolerance.

- **Back boards** support posture and apply pressure to the flanks and lower back, particularly after 360-degree liposuction. Without back support, patients often adopt hunched postures that may affect incision healing. Back boards help redistribute pressure and optimize silhouette shaping. These can be uncomfortable and sometimes foam pads are used as a substitute.
- **Foam pads** are soft inserts that help distribute compression evenly and reduce discomfort from garment seams. They are especially helpful for patients with sensitive skin or uneven swelling. Foam inserts prevent hard spots from developing under compression garments and should be worn as soon as swelling stabilizes, typically within the first 3–5 days post-op.
- **Genital pads** can be purchased or created using foam pads or menstrual pads. For women, the padding is placed more forward, from the opening of the vagina to the mons pubis. For men, a genital pad is placed under the scrotum. In both men and women, the pad should apply gentle pressure to swollen soft tissue between the legs. Genital pads help distribute compression evenly and reduce discomfort from fluid seeping into these regions from gravity.

Other adjuncts available include **chin straps** for neck lifts or facial liposuction, **arm compression sleeves** for brachioplasty or upper body liposuction, and **lateral support panels** for body sculpting procedures. Each serves a different purpose and must be introduced under professional guidance to avoid complications.

Patients are encouraged to check garment fit regularly. Swelling may reduce quickly in some areas while persisting in others, so garments should be adjusted or replaced to maintain appropriate compression without restricting circulation.

## Compression Garment Types and Styles

Compression garments for patients undergoing body contouring procedures come in a variety of types and styles designed to accommodate the diverse anatomical and functional needs of recovery. The selection of an appropriate compression garment can significantly influence patient comfort, contour outcomes, and compliance with post-operative care recommendations.

**Single-Wall vs. Double-Wall Fajas**

Single-wall fajas provide uniform compression using one layer of elasticized material. These are typically recommended for early stages of recovery (Stage 1) when swelling is at its peak and patients may need to remove and reapply garments frequently. They are easier to put on and more forgiving in areas prone to inflammation.

Double-wall fajas include an extra layer of compression fabric, offering firmer support. These are ideal for Stage 2 recovery (usually weeks 2–8), when more shaping is required and swelling has subsided. Double-wall fajas can help enhance contour definition, particularly in the waist and abdomen.

**Strap Design: Padded vs. Standard**

Shoulder straps come in various styles, with padded straps offering superior comfort, especially for patients with breast surgery or prolonged wear requirements. Padded straps help distribute pressure evenly and reduce indentation or chafing at the shoulders.

Adjustable straps, whether padded or not, are highly recommended for patients who may experience shifts in swelling or need to accommodate movement and posture changes during recovery.

**Zippers vs. Clips**

Fajas are typically secured using either a front zipper or 1-4 vertical rows of hook-and-eye clips. Zippers offer quicker application and removal but may create localized pressure points and can sometimes irritate healing skin or scars, especially if positioned over incision areas. Clips, on the other hand, offer greater adjustability, allowing patients to tighten or loosen the compression gradually as swelling reduces. For this reason, garments with at least three rows of hook-and-eye clips are preferred, particularly during the first four weeks of recovery. This adjustability supports improved contouring without needing to replace the entire garment as body measurements change.

**Going to the Bathroom**

To accommodate hygiene needs without removing the entire garment, fajas typically feature either a perineal zipper or an open crotch design. Zippers offer more coverage and discretion but may create pressure points if not aligned properly. Open crotch designs provide easier bathroom access, particularly for patients with limited mobility but the openings are often smaller, making it more difficult to keep clean.

Underwear is not typically worn under the compression garments to avoid having to remove the garment to use the bathroom.

Whether the faja has a zipper or open crotch, use of a female urinal device such as a handheld urinal or silicone funnel is highly recommended. These tools can improve hygiene and reduce frustration, especially during the early post-operative period when mobility is limited. Proper hygiene is essential to avoid infection, particularly for patients wearing garments 18–24 hours a day. Some fajas are treated with an antimicrobial element like silver, and they will tolerate washing on the delicate cycle in cold water.

Design and fit of the faja matters for comfort and to achieve recovery goals. Research by Tavares and Ferreira (2014) confirms that proper garment design significantly enhances patient compliance and reduces garment-related complications. Faja manufacturers continue to evolve styles with added convenience features, breathable fabrics, and odor-reducing linings to increase wearability.

## Abdominal Binders and Waist Trainers

Abdominal binders and waist trainers are two additional compression tools that offer distinct benefits during post-surgical recovery. While often used in conjunction with fajas or other garments, they can serve specific functions that enhance both comfort and aesthetic outcomes.

**Abdominal Binders**

Abdominal binders are wide, adjustable compression wraps made of elastic fabric. They are used in early stages of recovery after procedures such as liposuction, abdominoplasty (tummy tuck), C-section, or hernia repair. These binders offer support for abdominal muscles, reduce pain during movement, and help prevent fluid build-up (seromas).

Unlike fajas, binders are easy to adjust and remove. They are ideal for patients just after post-op when tight garments may not be tolerated. They can be used instead of fajas or used for lighter support, such as during sleep or low-activity.

**Waist Trainers**

Waist trainers are more rigid, contour-focused garments designed to cinch the waist and enhance hourglass shaping. While not intended for initial recovery, they may be introduced after the first 4–6 weeks once incisions are healed and swelling has reduced. Waist trainers can be worn over fajas to enhance shaping, particularly for patients undergoing procedures like liposuction or BBL.

Caution should be taken when using waist trainers, as overly tight or poorly fitted garments can impede breathing or compress internal organs. Their use should always be discussed with a provider or post-operative therapist.

Both abdominal binders and waist trainers may be worn for 3–4 months post-op, depending on patient goals and recovery progression. Consistent use supports continued contouring, reduces tissue laxity, and reinforces the surgical outcome. According to Lekic and Simunovic (2016), prolonged compression (up to 12 weeks) is associated with improved skin retraction and patient-reported satisfaction.

## Compression Socks and Compression Leggings

Compression socks and compression leggings are essential tools in post-operative recovery, especially for supporting circulation, minimizing the risk of deep vein thrombosis (DVT), and aiding in fluid management for the lower extremities. Their use is particularly important after procedures that involve prolonged bed rest, lower body surgeries, or systemic swelling.

**Compression Socks**

Compression socks apply graduated pressure to the feet and legs, which promotes venous return, reduces leg swelling, and helps prevent blood clots. Compression socks do their best work when used during times of movement – when the muscles can help pump the lymphatic fluid back up into the thigh or groin. Compression socks are frequently used after surgeries involving the abdomen, thighs, or even breasts, where limited mobility can increase the risk of circulatory issues. Socks are typically prescribed with a pressure rating measured in mmHg (millimeters of mercury):

- **15–20 mmHg**: Mild compression for everyday support
- **20–30 mmHg**: Moderate compression, often used in post-operative and mild varicose vein treatment
- **30–40 mmHg**: Firm compression, usually prescribed under physician supervision for more significant swelling or venous issues

A study by Rabe et al. (2010) found that compression therapy using socks with 20–30 mmHg significantly improved venous flow velocity and reduced the incidence of post-surgical thrombotic complications.

**Compression Leggings**

Compression leggings provide full-length pressure coverage to the lower body and are especially helpful for patients undergoing procedures like thigh lifts, lower body liposuction, or total body contouring. These garments support tissue shaping, help manage fluid retention, and reduce post-surgical discomfort in the legs, hips, and buttocks.

Leggings come in two main categories:

- **Circular knit leggings**, which are seamless and ideal for mild to moderate compression needs. They are typically more elastic and comfortable for all-day wear.
- **Flat or custom knit leggings**, which are more structured and used for patients requiring targeted compression (e.g., lymphedema or severe swelling). These are often custom-fitted and offer stronger support.

Compression leggings can be worn alone or layered over surgical garments like fajas during the mid to late phases of recovery. Regular assessment of fit is essential, as swelling reduction can make previously well-fitted garments loose, reducing their effectiveness.

Properly graded compression garments, including leggings, can reduce edema, promote lymphatic return, and enhance healing outcomes when used consistently throughout recovery [Damstra and Partsch (2013).

## Elastic Tape for Compression and Fibrosis Management

Elastic therapeutic taping, such as kinesiology tape, has emerged as a supportive adjunct in post-operative recovery, particularly for managing swelling, bruising, and fibrosis. Elastic tape is applied directly to the skin in specific patterns to facilitate lymphatic flow and support underlying tissue, without restricting range of motion.

**Benefits of Elastic Tape:**

Elastic tape gently lifts the skin, which can decompress the lymphatic channels and improve fluid drainage in areas affected by edema or hematoma. It is especially useful for patients who are unable to tolerate continuous pressure from garments or who need supplemental support in difficult-to-compress areas. A study by Lee et al. (2017) showed that kinesiology taping improved lymphatic return and reduced post-surgical swelling in patients following orthopedic and cosmetic procedures.

Taping also helps reduce fibrosis by improving blood and lymphatic circulation in localized areas of tissue stiffness. When applied over nodular or hardened regions, it can aid in softening texture, especially in conjunction with manual therapy or massage.

**Drawbacks and Considerations:**

While elastic taping has benefits, it is not a substitute for full-body compression garments. Its effects are localized and temporary, and taping requires skilled application to avoid skin irritation, blistering, or ineffective results. Incorrect placement or excessive tension can worsen skin trauma, especially in thin or fragile post-surgical skin.

Some patients may experience sensitivity to adhesives or allergic reactions to the tape's components. Additionally, the tape must be reapplied every 3–5 days and kept dry to prevent peeling or infection risk.

Elastic taping is best introduced by a trained lymphatic or post-operative therapist who understands the underlying anatomy and the patient's surgical plan. It can be particularly helpful during the transition out of 24/7 garment use or when tapering compression levels.

Compression Garments by Procedure and Timeline

| Garment Type | Common Surgeries | Week 1–2 | Week 3–4 | Week 5–8 |
|---|---|---|---|---|
| Faja (Stage 1) | BBL, liposuction, tummy tuck | Worn 24/7 | --- | --- |
| Faja (Stage 2) | BBL, liposuction, tummy tuck | --- | Worn 24/7 | Worn 24/7 |
| High-waisted leggings | Thigh lift, lower body lipo | Worn 24/7 | Worn 24/7 | Worn 12–18 hrs/day |
| Abdominal binder | Tummy tuck, C-section, hernia repair | Worn 24/7 | Worn 18-24 hrs/day | As Needed |
| Breast band | Breast aug/ reduction/lift | Worn as directed | Tapered use | As Needed |
| Sports bra (no underwire) | Breast surgeries, chest contouring | Worn 24/7 | Worn 24/7 | Worn 12–18 hrs/day |
| Chin strap | Neck lift, submental liposuction | Worn 24/7 | Worn nightly | As Needed for shaping |
| Arm sleeve | Brachioplasty, upper body lipo | Worn 24/7 | Worn 12–18 hrs/day | Worn as needed |

Always consult with your surgical team or lymphatic therapist before discontinuing use. Ill-fitting or premature removal of compression garments can contribute to swelling, contour irregularities, and discomfort.

It is recommended to gently wash and air-dry garments daily or every other day to maintain hygiene and elasticity.

# Bibliography


Association of periOperative Registered Nurses (AORN). (2020). Ambulation after surgery. AORN Guidelines. https://www.aorn.org/guidelines/about-aorn-guidelines

Al Mofeez, S., Al Abdulwahab, F., & Al Khalifah, M. (2021). Effectiveness of manual lymphatic drainage therapy on postoperative recovery: A systematic review. *Journal of Physical Therapy Science, 33*(4), 369–375.

Albertsmeier, M., et al. (2014). Enhanced recovery after surgery (ERAS) in gastrointestinal surgery. Surgery, 155(1), 9-14.

American Academy of Dermatology (AAD). (2020). Sunscreen FAQs. Retrieved from https://www.aad.org

American College of Obstetricians and Gynecologists. (2020). Postoperative care after gynecologic surgery. *ACOG Patient Education FAQ*. Retrieved from https://www.acog.org/womens-health/faqs/recovery-after-gynecologic-surgery

American College of Sports Medicine. (2021). Guidelines for Exercise Testing and Prescription (11th ed.).

Ammon, H.P. (2016). Boswellic acids and their role in chronic inflammatory diseases. Planta Medica, 82(14), 1123–1134.

Amsterdam, J.D., Li, Y., Soeller, I., Rockwell, K., Mao, J.J., & Shults, J. (2009). A randomized, double-blind, placebo-controlled trial of oral Matricaria recutita (chamomile) extract therapy for generalized anxiety disorder. Journal of Clinical Psychopharmacology, 29(4), 378–382.

Andersen, F. A. (2001). Final report on the safety assessment of Menthol and Menthone. International Journal of Toxicology, 20(Suppl 2), 61–73.

Ankri, S., & Mirelman, D. (1999). Antimicrobial properties of allicin from garlic. Microbes and Infection, 1(2), 125–129.

Apfel, C. C., et al. (2012). Postoperative nausea and vomiting. Anesthesiology, 117(2), 299–317.

Atiyeh, B. S., Janom, H. H., & Al-Amm, C. (2015). Evidence-based scar management: How to improve results with technique and technology. World Journal of Plastic Surgery, 4(1), 3-10.

Atiyeh, B. S., Janom, H. H., & Al-Amm, C. (2015). Evidence-based scar management: How to improve results with technique and technology. World Journal of Plastic Surgery, 4(1), 3–10.

Barnes, J., Anderson, L.A., Gibbons, S., & Phillipson, J.D. (2005). Echinacea species (Echinacea angustifolia (DC.) Hell., Echinacea pallida (Nutt.) Nutt., Echinacea purpurea (L.) Moench): a review of their chemistry, pharmacology, and clinical properties. Journal of Pharmacy and Pharmacology, 57(8), 929–954.

Basson, R., et al. (2010). Sexual function in women. Journal of Sexual Medicine, 7(1), 28–45.

Beard, J. L. (2001). Iron biology in immune function, muscle metabolism, and neuronal functioning. The Journal of Nutrition, 131(2), 568S–580S.

Bharucha, A. E., et al. (2013). American Gastroenterological Association medical position statement on constipation. Gastroenterology, 144(1), 211–217.

Bleakley, C. M., Glasgow, P., & Webb, M. J. (2012). The evidence base for the M.E.A.T. and R.I.C.E. guidelines in acute soft tissue injury management. British Journal of Sports Medicine.

Booth, S. L., Lichtenstein, A. H., O'Brien-Morse, M., McKeown, N. M., Wood, R. J., Saltzman, E., & Dawson-Hughes, B. (2003). Effects of vitamin K supplementation on bone loss in elderly men and women. The American Journal of Clinical Nutrition, 77(5), 1170-1175.

Brien, S., Lewith, G., Walker, A., Hicks, S. M., & Middleton, D. (2004). Bromelain as a treatment for osteoarthritis: a review of clinical studies. Phytomedicine, 11(7-8), 585-593.

Brinkhaus, B., Lindner, M., Schuppan, D., & Hahn, E.G. (2000). Chemical, pharmacological, and clinical profile of the East Asian medical plant Centella asiatica. Phytomedicine, 7(5), 427–448.

Brosseau, L., et al. (2004). Effects of exercise on physical function and quality of life in patients with fibromyalgia. Journal of Rheumatology, 31(6), 1131–1140.

Brown, R. P., & Gerbarg, P. L. (2005). Sudarshan Kriya Yogic breathing in the treatment of stress, anxiety, and depression: Part II, clinical applications and guidelines. *Journal of Alternative and Complementary Medicine, 11*(4), 711–717.

Buvanendran, A., & Kroin, J. S. (2009). Multimodal analgesia for controlling acute postoperative pain. Current Opinion in Anesthesiology, 22(5), 588-593.

Børsheim, E., Tipton, K. D., Wolf, S. E., & Wolfe, R. R. (2008). Essential amino acids and muscle protein recovery after resistance exercise. The American Journal of Physiology-Endocrinology and Metabolism, 283(4), E648-E657.

Calder, P. C. (2013). Omega-3 polyunsaturated fatty acids and inflammatory processes: Nutrition or pharmacology? British Journal of Clinical Pharmacology, 75(3), 645-662.

Carli, F., et al. (2010). Surgical prehabilitation in patients with cancer: State-of-the-science and recommendations for future research from a panel of subject matter experts.

Physical Medicine and Rehabilitation Clinics of North America, 21(1), 91-104.

Carr, A. C., & Maggini, S. (2017). Vitamin C and immune function. Nutrients, 9(11), 1211.

Carson, C.F., Hammer, K.A., & Riley, T.V. (2006). Melaleuca alternifolia (Tea Tree) oil: A review of antimicrobial and other medicinal properties. Clinical Microbiology Reviews, 19(1), 50–62.

Cereda, E., Klersy, C., Serioli, M., Crespi, A., & D'Andrea, F. (2015). A nutritional formula enriched with arginine, zinc, and antioxidants for the healing of pressure ulcers: A randomized trial. *Annals of Internal Medicine, 162*(3), 167–174.

Chaudhry, M. A., Shabbir, A., & Ali, A. (2020). Surgical drains: Indications, types, and complications. *Cureus, 12*(4), e7541.

Cheville, A. L., McGarvey, C. L., Petrek, J. A., Russo, S. A., Taylor, M. E., & Thiadens, S. R. (2001). Lymphedema management. Cancer, 92(4 Suppl), 977–987.

Chia, H. L., Tay, E. Y., Phua, T. C., & Lim, T. C. (2015). Postoperative scar management following rhytidectomy: A review of strategies to optimize results. Journal of Cosmetic and Laser Therapy, 17(1), 1–7.

Cho, Y. S., Jeon, J. H., Hong, A., Yang, H. T., Yim, H., & Cho, Y. S. (2014). The effect of scar massage on hypertrophic scar after burn: A randomized controlled trial. Burns, 40(8), 1515–1520.

Courneya, K. S., & Friedenreich, C. M. (2007). Physical activity and cancer control. Current Opinion in Oncology, 19(4), 295–301.

Cárdenas-Camarena, L., Durán, H., & Robles-Cervantes, J. A. (2015). Postoperative fibrosis in liposuction and gluteal fat grafting: Diagnosis, prevention, and treatment. Aesthetic Plastic Surgery, 39(6), 901–909.

Daily, J. W., Yang, M., & Park, S. (2016). Efficacy of turmeric extracts and curcumin for alleviating the symptoms of joint arthritis: a systematic review and meta-analysis of randomized clinical trials. Journal of Ethnopharmacology, 175, 120-130.

Damstra, R. J., & Partsch, H. (2013). Prospective, randomized, controlled trial comparing the effectiveness of Velcro adjustable compression devices with compression bandages in the initial treatment of leg lymphedema. Journal of Vascular Surgery: Venous and Lymphatic Disorders, 1(1), 13–19.

de Luis, D. A., et al. (2021). Nutritional status and postoperative outcomes. Clinical Nutrition, 40(4), 2027-2034.

Dubois, B., & Esculier, J. F. (2020). Soft-tissue injuries simply need PEACE and LOVE. British Journal of Sports Medicine, 54(2), 72–73. https://doi.org/10.1136/bjsports-2019-101253

Draelos, Z. D. (2013). The multifunctional role of niacinamide in dermatology. Cutis, 92(5), 237–241.

Eaves, F. F., Rohrich, R. J., & Sykes, J. M. (2013). Finding the right surgeon: Why board certification matters. Plastic and Reconstructive Surgery, 132(6), 1377-1382.

Ebner, F., Heller, A., Rippke, F., & Tausch, I. (2002). Topical use of dexpanthenol in skin disorders. American Journal of Clinical Dermatology, 3(6), 427–433.

Ernst, E., & Pittler, M. H. (2000). Efficacy of ginger for nausea and vomiting: A meta-analysis. British Journal of Anaesthesia, 84(3), 367–371.

Evans, D. C., Corkins, M. R., Malone, A., Miller, S., Mogensen, K. M., Guenter, P., & Jensen, G. L. (2020). The use of visceral proteins as nutrition markers: An ASPEN position paper. *Nutrition in Clinical Practice, 35*(1), 29–48.

Field, T. (2014). Massage therapy research review. Complementary Therapies in Clinical Practice, 20(4), 224–229.

Fowler, C. J., et al. (2008). Postoperative urinary retention and voiding dysfunction. British Journal of Urology International, 101(1), 11–15.

Franklin, M. E., et al. (2008). Integration of physical therapy and massage therapy in post-surgical care. Archives of Physical Medicine and Rehabilitation, 89(12), 2217–2223.

Fruhstorfer, B. H., Malata, C. M., & Trott, S. A. (2013). Wound healing and scar management in plastic surgery. British Journal of Surgery, 100(2), 188–200.

Földi, M., Strößenreuther, R. H., & Földi, E. (2019). Lymphatic drainage and its role in post-surgical edema reduction. Journal of Dermatological Treatment.

Gurtner, G. C., Werner, S., Barrandon, Y., & Longaker, M. T. (2011). Wound repair and regeneration. Nature, 453(7193), 314-321.

Hashemi, S.A., Madani, S.A., & Abediankenari, S. (2015). The review on properties of Aloe vera in healing of cutaneous wounds. BioMed Research International, 2015, Article ID 714216. https://doi.org/10.1155/2015/714216

Hewlings, S.J., & Kalman, D.S. (2017). Curcumin: A review of its effects on human health. Foods, 6(10), 92.

Hidalgo, D. A., & Spector, J. A. (2010). Surgical strategies for optimizing body contouring outcomes. Clinics in Plastic Surgery, 37(3), 451–462.

Hilde, G., et al. (2016). Effect of pelvic floor muscle training for women with pelvic organ prolapse. BMJ, 354, i3729.

Hildebrandt, C., et al. (2003). The effectiveness of manual lymph drainage in patients with orthopedic surgery. Journal of Manual & Manipulative Therapy, 11(3), 121–127.

Honigman, R. J., Phillips, K. A., & Castle, D. J. (2004). A review of psychosocial outcomes for patients seeking cosmetic surgery. Plastic and Reconstructive Surgery, 113(4), 1229–1237.

Iannitti, T., Morales-Medina, J.C., Bellavite, P., Rottigni, V., & Palmieri, B. (2016). Effectiveness and safety of Arnica montana in post-surgical setting, pain, and inflammation. American Journal of Therapeutics, 23(1), e184–e197.

Jacka, F. N., et al. (2017). The role of diet in mental health. The Lancet Psychiatry, 4(3), 271-281.

Kang, S., Voorhees, J. J., & Chung, J. H. (2005). Topical retinoids and their role in photoaging. Dermatologic Therapy, 18(5), 253–264.

Kiecolt-Glaser, J. K., Page, G. G., Marucha, P. T., MacCallum, R. C., & Glaser, R. (2005). Psychological influences on surgical recovery: Perspectives from psychoneuroimmunology. American Psychologist, 60(3), 240–251.

Kim, D. Y., Jeong, E. C., & Lee, D. W. (2015). Effect of closed-suction drainage in preventing seroma formation after breast surgery: A meta-analysis. *Annals of Surgical Treatment and Research, 89*(6), 290–297.

Kim, J. H., Park, J. H., & Lee, Y. S. (2018). Effects of scar massage on joint range of motion and pain after total knee arthroplasty: A randomized controlled trial. Journal of Physical Therapy Science, 30(8), 1043–1046.

Kim, Y. H., et al. (2011). Effectiveness of compression garments in postoperative recovery: A meta-analysis. Annals of Plastic Surgery, 67(4), 357–364.

Kingsberg, S. A., et al. (2013). Vulvovaginal atrophy in postmenopausal women: Impact and treatment. Journal of Sexual Medicine, 10(7), 1790–1799.

Klinger, M., Caviggioli, F., Klinger, F. M., Maione, L., & Lisa, A. (2018). Emotional impact and perception of the self-image in patients after cosmetic surgery. Aesthetic Plastic Surgery, 42(4), 1210–1216.

Kubler-Ross, E., & Kessler, D. (2005). On Grief and Grieving: Finding the Meaning of Grief Through the Five Stages of Loss. Scribner.

Kuipers, S., Cannegieter, S. C., Middeldorp, S., Robyn, L., & Büller, H. R. (2011). The risk of venous thrombosis after air travel. Annals of Internal Medicine, 154(7), 459-467.

Kulber, D. A., Bacilious, N., Peters, E. D., & Peters, W. (2009). Sensory recovery after breast augmentation. Plastic and Reconstructive Surgery, 123(5), 1235–1242.

Lang, H., Meyer, L., Peter, M., & Martens, C. (2017). Hydration and its effects on wound healing in post-surgical recovery. Aesthetic Surgery Journal, 37(4), 480-486.

Leduc, O., et al. (2009). Manual lymph drainage and therapeutic patient education in breast cancer-related lymphedema. Journal of Lymphoedema, 4(1), 18–24.

Lee, J. H., Yoo, W. G., & Lee, K. S. (2017). Effects of kinesiology taping on lymphatic drainage and fibrosis reduction after surgery. Journal of Physical Therapy Science, 29(8), 1394–1397.

Lee, K. C., & Mun, G. H. (2013). The efficacy of early postoperative scar management: A systematic review of scar-related studies in plastic surgery. Annals of Plastic Surgery, 71(6), 673–679.

Lee, S. H., & Hwang, K. (2017). The efficacy of manual lymphatic drainage in postoperative recovery after plastic surgery: A systematic review. *Aesthetic Plastic Surgery, 41*(5), 1090–1096.

Lekic, N., & Simunovic, V. (2016). The use of compression

therapy after aesthetic surgery: A clinical review. Journal of Aesthetic Nursing, 5(7), 318–324.

Lever, E., et al. (2019). Systematic review of dietary interventions for the management of functional constipation in adults. American Journal of Clinical Nutrition, 110(5), 1102–1110.

Levi, B., Kraft, C. T., Shapiro, A., Trinh, N. T., Dore, C., & Levine, J. P. (2018). The association of pre-operative preparation with recovery after surgery: A systematic review. Journal of Surgical Research, 222, 123-133.

Levine, M., et al. (2014). Perioperative management of antithrombotic therapy: Antithrombotic Therapy and Prevention of Thrombosis, 9th ed: American College of Chest Physicians Evidence-Based Clinical Practice Guidelines. Chest, 141(2_suppl), e326S-e350S.

Lieber, C. S. (2004). Alcohol, nutrient metabolism, and complications of alcohol abuse. Annals of Internal Medicine, 139(8), 603-614.

Lieber, C. S. (2004). Relationships between nutrition, alcohol use, and liver disease. New England Journal of Medicine, 350(17), 1705-1714.

Lin, P.-H., Sermersheim, M., Li, H., Lee, P. H. U., Steinberg, S. M., & Ma, J. (2017). Zinc in wound healing modulation. *Nutrients, 10*(1), 16.

Liu, C., Feng, X., Li, Q., Wang, Y., Li, Q., Hua, M., ... & Chen, Y. (2014). High dietary sugar intake and increased inflammation. The American Journal of Clinical Nutrition, 99(3), 624-632.

Lobo, D. N., Macafee, D. A., & Allison, S. P. (2006). How perioperative fluid balance influences postoperative outcomes. *Best Practice & Research Clinical Anaesthesiology, 20*(3), 439–455.

Lodén, M., & Maibach, H. I. (2009). Treatment of dry skin syndrome: The art and science of moisturizing. Springer Science & Business Media.

Lustig, R. H., Schmidt, L. A., & Brindis, C. D. (2012). The toxic truth about sugar. *Nature, 482*(7383), 27–29.

Mainil, T., et al. (2017). Medical tourism and its impact on healthcare systems. Global Health Journal.

Malcolm, R., & Tallian, K. (2017). Essential oils in the treatment of anxiety and depression: A systematic review of the literature. Mental Health Clinician, 7(4), 147–155.

Mangram, A. J., Horan, T. C., Pearson, M. L., Silver, L. C., & Jarvis, W. R. (1999). Guideline for prevention of surgical site infection, 1999. *Infection Control and Hospital Epidemiology, 20*(4), 250–278.

Manuskiatti, W., & Fitzpatrick, R. E. (2002). Treatment response of keloidal and hypertrophic sternotomy scars: Comparison among intralesional corticosteroid, 585-nm flashlamp-pumped pulsed-dye laser, and combined treatment. *Archives of Dermatology, 138*(9), 1149–1155.

Matarasso, A., & Wallach, S. G. (2005). Liposuction. Plastic and Reconstructive Surgery, 115(2), 69e–85e.

Matarasso, A., et al. (2014). Abdominoplasty: Classic principles and techniques. Plastic and Reconstructive Surgery, 134(4), 709–717.

McNeely, M. L., et al. (2010). Exercise interventions for upper-limb dysfunction due to breast cancer treatment. Cochrane Database of Systematic Reviews, Issue 6.

Molan, P.C. (2001). Honey as a topical antibacterial agent for treatment of infected wounds. World Wide Wounds, 2001. Retrieved from http://www.worldwidewounds.com/2001/november/Molan/honey-as-topical-agent.html

Moore, F. A., Phillips, S. M., McClain, C. J., Patel, J. J., & Martindale, R. G. (2014). Nutrition support for persistent inflammation, immunosuppression, and catabolism syndrome. Nutrition in Clinical Practice, 29(3), 306-313.

Mortimer, P. S., & Rockson, S. G. (2014). New developments in clinical aspects of lymphatic disease. Journal of Clinical Investigation, 124(3), 915–921.

Moser, D. A., et al. (2019). Psychological preparation for surgery. Journal of Clinical Psychology in Medical Settings, 26(1), 54-62.

Mustoe, T. A., Cooter, R. D., Gold, M. H., Hobbs, R., Ramelet, A. A., Shakespeare, P. G., Stella, M., Téot, L., Wood, F. M., & Ziegler, U. E. (2002). International clinical recommendations on scar management. Plastic and Reconstructive Surgery, 110(2), 560–571.

Nicolle, L. E. (2014). Catheter-associated urinary tract infections. Antimicrobial Resistance and Infection Control, 3(1), 23.

North, B. B., Oldham, M. J., & Gannon, M. J. (2020). A review of menstrual cup use and safety: Implications for post-surgical and gynecologic care. *Journal of Women's Health*, *29*(8), 1038–1044.

O'Brien, L., & Jones, D. J. (2013). Silicone gel sheeting for preventing and treating hypertrophic and keloid scars. Cochrane Database of Systematic Reviews, 9, CD003826.

Ouwehand, A. C., Kirjavainen, P. V., Shortt, C., & Salminen, S. (2002). Probiotics: Mechanisms and established effects. International Dairy Journal, 9(1), 43-52.

Ouwehand, A. C., et al. (2002). Probiotic and other functional microbes: From markets to mechanisms. Current Opinion in Biotechnology, 13(5), 483–487.

O'Brien, L., & Jones, D. J. (2013). Silicone gel sheeting for preventing and treating hypertrophic and keloid scars. Cochrane Database of Systematic Reviews, 9, CD003826.

Pannucci, C. J., Antony, A. K., Wilkins, E. G., & Kim, J. Y. S. (2012). The impact of drain duration on surgical-site infection in prosthetic breast reconstruction. *Plastic and Reconstructive Surgery, 129*(4), 913–921.

Pedersen, B. K., & Saltin, B. (2015). Exercise as medicine: Evidence for prescribing exercise as therapy in 26 different chronic diseases. Scandinavian Journal of Medicine & Science in Sports, 25(S3), 1-72.

Phillips, S. M. (2016). Dietary protein for athletes: From requirements to metabolic advantage. Applied Physiology, Nutrition, and Metabolism, 41(5), 498-503.

Phillips, S. M. (2016). The impact of protein quality on the promotion of resistance exercise-induced changes in muscle mass. Advances in Nutrition, 7(3), 511-519.

Pludowski, P., Holick, M. F., Pilz, S., Wagner, C. L., Hollis, B. W., Grant, W. B., Shoenfeld, Y., Lerchbaum, E., Llewellyn, D. J., Kienreich, K., & Soni, M. (2013). Vitamin D effects on musculoskeletal health, immunity, autoimmunity, cardiovascular disease, cancer, fertility, pregnancy, dementia and mortality, a review of recent evidence. *Autoimmunity Reviews, 12*(10), 976–989.Popkin et al.. (2010). *Title missing*. Source missing.

Popkin, B. M., et al. (2010). Water, hydration, and health. Nutrition Reviews, 68(8), 439–458.

Porras-Reyes, B. H., Lewis, W. H., Roman, J., Simchowitz, L., & Mustoe, T. A. (1993). Enhancement of wound healing by the alkaloid taspine defining mechanism of action. *Proceedings of the Society for Experimental Biology and Medicine, 203*(1), 18–25.Practice Committee of the ASRM. (2015). *Title missing*. Source missing.

Practice Committee of the American Society for Reproductive Medicine. (2015). Committee Opinion: Menstrual health post-surgery. Fertility and Sterility, 104(1), 54–58.

Preethi, K.C., & Kuttan, R. (2009). Wound healing activity of flower extract of Calendula officinalis. Journal of Basic and Clinical Physiology and Pharmacology, 20(1), 73–80.

Rabe, E., Partsch, H., Hafner, J., Lattimer, C., Mosti, G., Neumann, M., & Urbanek, T. (2010). Indications for medical compression stockings in venous and lymphatic disorders: An evidence-based consensus statement. Phlebology, 25(4), 138–145.

Rawlings, A. V., & Harding, C. R. (2004). Moisturization and skin barrier function. Dermatologic Therapy, 17(Suppl 1), 43–48.

Reavey, P. L., Klassen, A. F., Cano, S. J., Pusic, A. L., & Scott, A. M. (2011). Measuring patient-reported outcomes in cosmetic and reconstructive breast surgery: A systematic review of validated instruments. Plastic and Reconstructive Surgery, 127(1), 181–191.

Reid, G., et al. (2001). Probiotics in the prevention of urinary tract infections and vaginal health. American Journal of Clinical Nutrition, 73(2), 437S–443S.

Reid, K., O'Neill, S., O'Sullivan, T., et al. (2015). Pain management after surgery: A review of current strategies. Journal of Clinical Medicine, 4(3), 240-256.

Rohrich, R. J., Beran, S. J., Kenkel, J. M., & Adams, W. P. (2006). Extending the role of open suction-assisted lipectomy: A 15-year experience. Plastic and Reconstructive Surgery, 117(7), 233–239.

Rohrich, R. J., Sorokin, E. S., & Brown, S. A. (2008). In search of improved outcomes in body contouring surgery: A review of the literature. Plastic and Reconstructive Surgery, 121(3), 698–706.

Rondanelli, M., Miccono, A., Lamburghini, S., Avanzato, I., Riva, A., Allegrini, P., ... & Perna, S. (2020). Food pyramid for subjects with chronic pain: foods and dietary constituents as anti-inflammatory and antioxidant agents. Nutrients, 12(6), 1676. https://doi.org/10.3390/nu12061676

Rosanoff, A., Weaver, C. M., & Rude, R. K. (2012). Suboptimal magnesium status in the United States: Are the health consequences underestimated? *Nutrition Reviews, 70*(3), 153–164.Santa Mina, D., Clarke, H., Ritvo, P., Leung, Y. W., Matthew, A. G., Katz, J., ... & Alibhai, S. M. (2014). Effect of total-body prehabilitation on postoperative outcomes: A systematic review and meta-analysis. Physiotherapy, 100(3), 196-207.

Sarwer, D. B., & Crerand, C. E. (2004). Body image and cosmetic medical treatments. Body Image, 1(1), 99–111.

Sarwer, D. B., Wadden, T. A., Pertschuk, M. J., & Whitaker, L. A. (2005). Body image dissatisfaction and body dysmorphic disorder in 100 cosmetic surgery patients. Plastic and Reconstructive Surgery, 116(5), 1336–1340.

Schellenberger, M. D., et al. (2007). Soft tissue therapy following orthopedic surgery. Journal of Bodywork and Movement Therapies, 11(3), 221–229.

Shelbourne, K. D., & Nitz, P. (2012). Accelerated rehabilitation after ACL reconstruction. American Journal of Sports Medicine, 20(3), 309–315.

Slavin, J. (2013). Dietary fiber and gut health. Current Opinion in Clinical Nutrition & Metabolic Care, 16(5), 624–629.

Sorensen, L. T. (2012). Wound healing and infection in surgery: The clinical impact of smoking and smoking cessation: A systematic review and meta-analysis. Archives of Surgery, 147(4), 373-383.

Stephenson, K., et al. (2020). The role of vitamin A and beta-carotene in immune function and inflammation. Nutrients, 12(5), 1520.

Strauch, B., Yu, H. L., & Vatsia, S. K. (2008). Mechanisms of seroma formation: Facts and myths. Plastic and Reconstructive Surgery, 122(3), 892–898.

Stuckey, H. L., & Nobel, J. (2010). The connection between art, healing, and public health: A review of current literature. American Journal of Public Health, 100(2), 254–263.

Suami, H., Scaglioni, M. F., & Wong, C. (2017). Changes in lymphatic drainage pathways following mastectomy and abdominoplasty: Evaluation using indocyanine green lymphography. Plastic and Reconstructive Surgery, 139(3), 761e–769e.

Tan, J., & Liu, J. (2018). The role of massage therapy in scar management: A systematic review. Journal of Dermatological Treatment, 29(7), 619-627.

Tanna, N., & Patel, P. K. (2017). Revision aesthetic surgery: Concepts and strategies. Facial Plastic Surgery Clinics of North America, 25(3), 367–377.

Tavares, C., & Ferreira, M. C. (2014). The importance of compression garments and foam in post-operative care after liposuction and lipoabdominoplasty. Aesthetic Surgery Journal, 34(4), 547–552.

Weimann, A., et al. (2017). ESPEN guidelines on clinical nutrition. Clinical Nutrition, 36(3), 623-650.

World Health Organization. (2016). Global guidelines for the prevention of surgical site infection. Geneva: WHO.

Zeidan, F., Johnson, S. K., Diamond, B. J., David, Z., & Goolkasian, P. (2011). Mindfulness meditation improves cognition: Evidence of brief mental training. Consciousness and Cognition, 19(2), 597-605.

von Soest, T., Kvalem, I. L., Roald, H. E., & Skolleborg, K. C. (2006). The effects of cosmetic surgery on body image, self-esteem, and psychological problems. Plastic and Reconstructive Surgery, 120(7), 1827–1835.

# About the Author

**Kevin Rebman, BCTMB, AAS, BA, MS, NREMT**, is a clinical manual soft tissue therapist, educator, and the founder of Return to Play Institute, LLC, a leading recovery-focused soft tissue therapy practice in Minneapolis, MN. Kevin blends clinical precision with compassionate care, specializing in post-operative healing, lymphatic health, neuromuscular therapy, athlete performance improvement, and scar tissue management.

Driven by a passion for results-backed recovery, Kevin bridges the worlds of science and human connection. His mission: to empower patients with the knowledge, techniques, and confidence they need to take charge of their healing journey.

As chief myotherapist, Kevin is board-certified in massage and bodywork, holds degrees from the University of Wisconsin–Green Bay, Aspen University, and Northwestern Health Sciences University, where he earned his AAS in Clinical Massage Therapy. He is also certified in perinatal massage, lymphatic drainage, complete decongestive therapy, oncology massage, and neuromuscular therapy. Outside the clinic, he serves as an Emergency Medical Technician and works youth sporting events—always ready to lend a hand where healing is needed most.

Whether he's working one-on-one with clients, training professionals, or advocating for higher standards in post-surgical care, Kevin remains at the forefront of a growing movement to redefine what good recovery can look like. For appointments, speaking opportunities, or training, Kevin can be reached through the clinic www.returntoplayinstitute.com.

www.ingramcontent.com/pod-product-compliance
Lightning Source LLC
LaVergne TN
LVHW090405210926
848480LV00002B/455